Comparative Embryology of the Domestic Cat

A short illustrated Embryology for veterinary students

Clemens Knospe

Copyright © 2013 Clemens Knospe

2nd edition 2015

All rights reserved.

ISBN: 1494304597
ISBN-13: 978-1494304591

PREFACE

Embryology is not only important for the understanding of the basic principles of development, but also for the understanding of gross anatomical and histological structures in the adult. It is important for many aspects of theriogenology, the diagnosis of cyclic stages, infertility and congenital malformations. Additionally embryology is the basis for advanced studies like embryo transfer, invitro-fertilization and cloning. Therefore this booklet has a new concept with less text but many original pictures to help reading experimental, embryological findings. All terms are according to the 2nd edition of the Nomina Embryologica Veterinaria (NEV). Low magnification of the microscopic pictures is marked by x, high magnification is marked by xxx.

Munich, December 2013 and July 2015

CONTENTS

1	Gametogenesis	9
2	Early Development	22
3	Fetogenesis and Histogenesis	35
4	Circulatory System	36
5	Digestive Apparatus	45
6	Respiratory Apparatus	56
7	Urogenital Apparatus	61
8	Nervous System	70
9	Skin and Derivatives	87
10	Locomotive Apparatus	91
	References and Index	100

INTRODUCTION

Embryology is the study of growth and differentiation, the development of a new organism. According to the theory of Weisman development is a cyclic event in the eternal life of germ cells. In their diploid somatic stage they are part of the body and in their free haploid stage they fuse during fertilization to reformat, remix their genes and start again to produce an individual somatic line, which develops into a new body as carrier for the germ cells. From this view development is divided into two phases: the gametogenesis (proontogenesis) in the adult organism with the transformation of the germ cells to gametes, and the ontogenesis, the development of the mortal body, starting with the fertilization. The ontogeny has three main periods: the preembryonal, the embryonal and the fetal period, which are subdivided by the NEV for comparative reasons into 15 phases. These are further subdivided into different stages in different species. The development of the domestic cat has 22 stages (Knospe, 2002). The preembryonal period is the primitive development with the morphogenesis, the embryonal period is the development of organs and tissues and the fetal period is the differentiation of organs and tissues (histogenesis). After birth the development continues with the postnatal and prepubertal period. According to Haeckel's theory of recapitulation even more embryology repeats the evolutionary development, the phylogeny.

Gametogenesis

Gametogenesis or Proontogenesis is the production of the gametes during spermatogenesis and oogenesis, the development of the male and female germ cells in three main phases: the separation of the primordial germ cells and their migration to the gonad, the specific proliferation up the puberty, and the specific differentiation up to fertile germ cells.

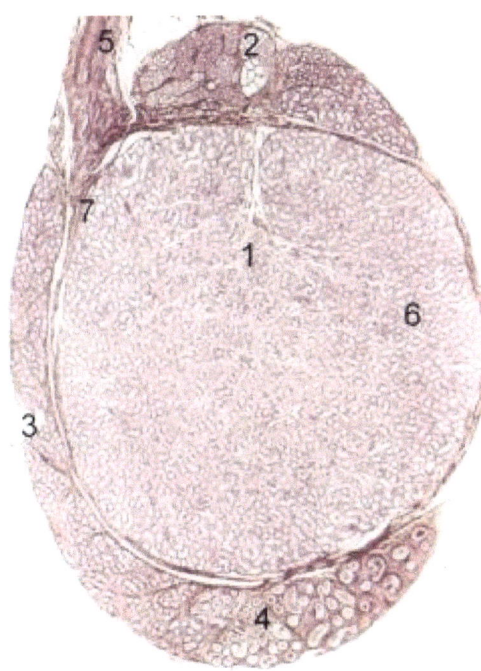

Fig.1: Testis, cat, xHE (x=low primary magnification, HE= Hematoxylin-Eosin stain): 1 mediastinum, 2 head, 3 body, 4 and tail of epididymis, 5 funiculus, 6 lobuli with tubuli seminiferi.

Spermatogenesis

The primordial germ cells in the testis form spermatogonia that proliferate throughout the breeding period of male animals, depending on the appropriate androgen stimulus. During sexual maturation (puberty) the process of the development of fertile sperm cells, called spermatogenesis, is started in the male gonad. Spermatogenesis can be subdivided into three phases: spermatocytogenesis, during which the spermatogonia develop into spermatocytes, meiosis, the maturation division of diploid spermatocytes into haploid spermatids, and spermiogenesis, the process of transformation of spermatids into spermatozoa. The duration of the process is approximately

30 days in boars, 35-40 days in dogs and cats, 40-50 days in bulls, rams, stallions, and 74 days in men. Another 2 - 3 weeks may be required for the passage through the epididymis. The ejaculate or semen is formed by a mixture of spermatozoa with secretions from the accessory glands, which serves as dilution, nutrition and activator of the spermatozoa.

Spermatocytogenesis

Spermatogonia proliferate mitotically to form A and I-spermatogonia. Type A is a large cell next to the basal lamina and will continue to proliferate, while I-spermatogonia are smaller, shift upward and divide into B-spermatogonia. The type B-spermatogonia are darker, connected by cytoplasmatic processes and divide to connected preleptotene spermatocytes, which move to the adluminal tubular compartment across the intercellular junctions between the sertoli cells. In these preleptotene cells the DNA is replicated to form two sister chromatids of each chromosome.

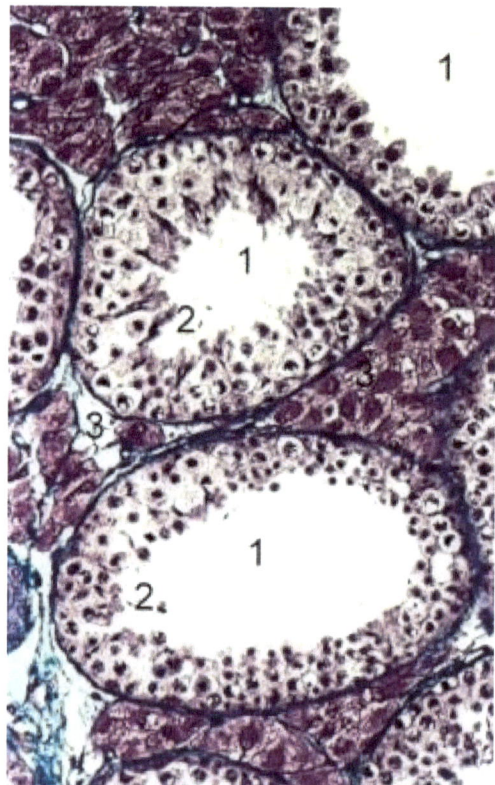

Fig.2: Testis, boar, xxGRA (xx= medium primary magnification, GRA=special trichrome stain): 1 tubuli, 2 seminal epithelium, 3 Leydig cells.

Meiosis

During meiosis primary spermatocytes undergo two successive nuclear divisions, resulting in four haploid spermatids. Primary spermatocytes are the largest tubular cells in the intermediate location of the spermatic tubules. The proleptotene primary spermatocytes enter the prophase of the first maturation division. During the leptotene stage their chromosomes become coiled to thin strands. In the zygotene stage homologous chromosomes pair to form tetrads of chromatids. Exchange in the so called synaptonemal complexes are made during this stage. In the pachytene stage this is completed as crossing over. During diplotaen the chromatids start to split only attached by chiasmata. Then the diakinesis ends the prophase, chromosomes shorten, separate, and the subsequent metaphase, anaphase and telophase ends the first division with two daughter secondary spermatocytes having a dyade of two chromatids. The secondary spermatocytes occur only for a short time. They undergo the second maturation division, similar to a normal mitotic division, in which the centromers divide and the chromatids are distributed to each of the spermatids resulting from this division.

Spermiogenesis

Spermiogenesis is the process where interconnected clones of spermatids undergo a metamorphosis to form highly differentiated spermatozoa in four phases:

a. During the **Golgi phase** the proacrosomal granules form the acrosomal vesicle.

b. During the **cap phase** the acrosomal vesicle forms the head cap in an eccentric position, and the centrioles assemble at the caudal pole. From the distal centriol a flagellum is outgrowing.

c. During the **acrosomal phase** nucleus and cytoplasm start to elongate, rotating the tail to the lumen. Nuclear DNA is denser packed by special basic proteins (protamines) instead of normal histones. The mitochondria become concentrated around the proximal part of the flagellum which forms the middle piece of the spermatozoa.

d. During the **maturation phase** nuclear condensation and formation of all parts are completed. Cyctoplasmatic bridges are disconnected, the excess of cytoplasm is detached as residual body, phagocytosed by sertoli cells, and the sperm cells are released.

Tubulus Stage

Several spermatogenic series are started all 4 hours at the same level of a given tubule. As all descends develop synchronously, successive cell generations form a typical pattern, a typical composition of the seminal epithelium at that tubule section, called a tubular stage. These stages are continuing through the tubules in one direction forming a wave of differentiating cells along a tubule. There are different approaches to differentiate the different tubule pictures of different species into a more or less number of stages. Systems with 4 (bull, boar) up to 14 (rat) stages exist, making the comparision difficult. The following comparative system of 6 stages is covering all species:

I Postcytokinesis Stage   **II Prespermiation Stage**

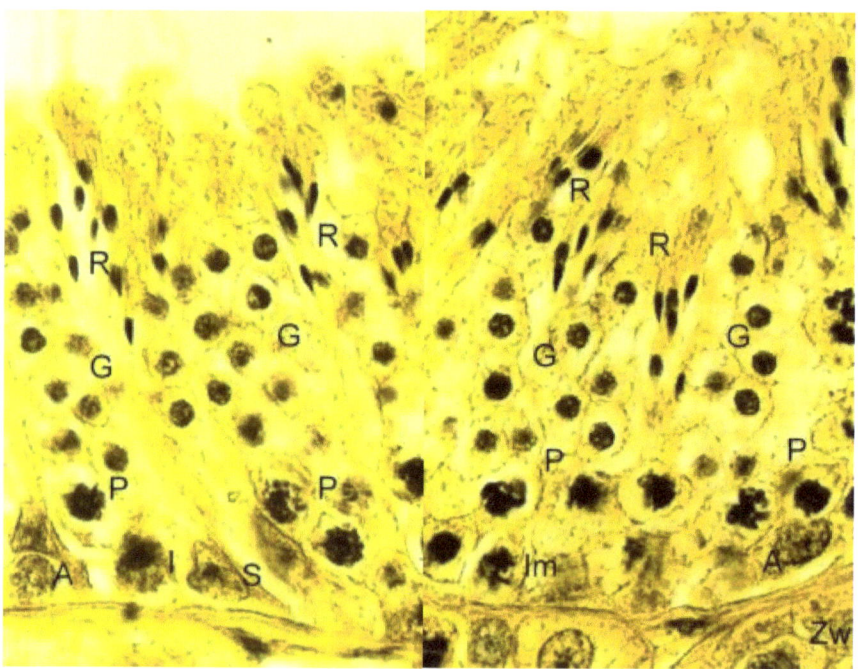

Fig.3 (left side): Seminal epithelium, cat, xxxEH (xxx= high primary magnification, EH=iron-hematoxylin stain): postcytokinese stage with A-spermatogonia (A), I-spermatogonia (I), sertoli cell (S), pachytene spermatocytes (P), Golgi spermatids (G), maturation spermatids (R).

Fig.4 (right side): Seminal epithelium, cat, xxxEH: prespermiation stage with A-spermatogonia (A), I-spermatogonia (I), pachytene spermatocytes (P), Golgi spermatids (G), maturation spermatides (R).

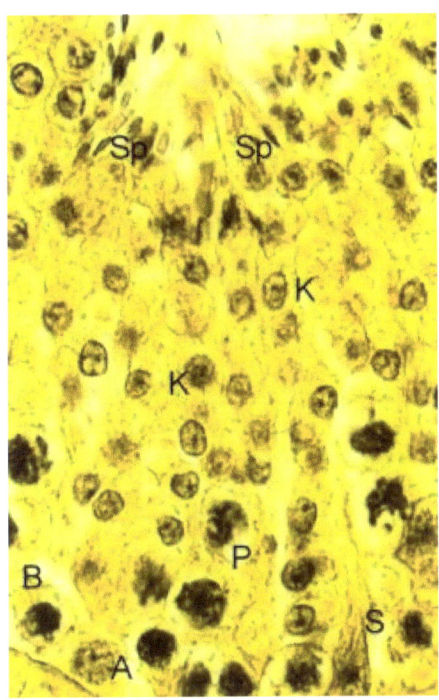

III Spermiation Stage

Fig.5: Seminal epithelium, cat, xxxEH: spermiation stage with A-spermatogonia (A), B-spermatogonia (B), sertoli cell (S), pachytene spermatocytes (P), cap spermatids (K), sperm cells (Sp).

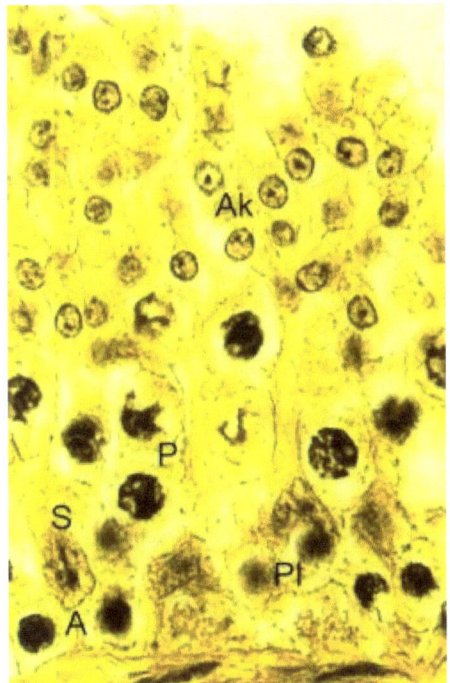

IV Postspermiation Stage

Fig.6: Seminal epithelium, cat, xxxEH: postspermiation stage with A-spermatogonia (A), preleptotene spermatocytes (PL), pachytene spermatocytes (P), akrosomal spermatids (Ak).

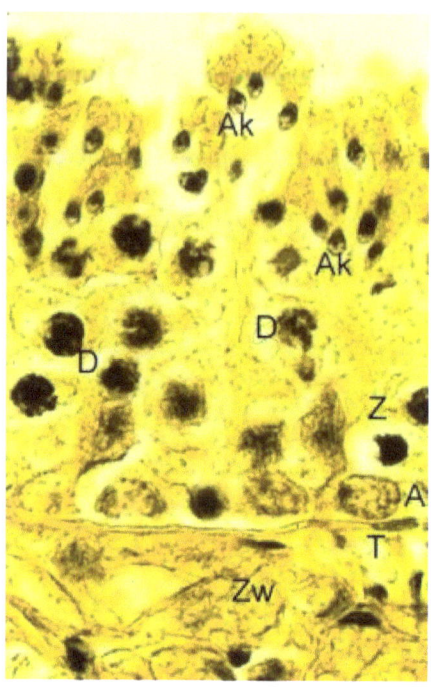

V Precytokinesis Stage

Fig.7: Seminal epithelium, cat, xxxEH: precytokinesis stage with A-spermatogia (A), diplotene spermatozytes (D), zygotene spermatozytes (Z), akrosomal spermatides (Ak), peritubular cell (T), Leydig cells (Zw).

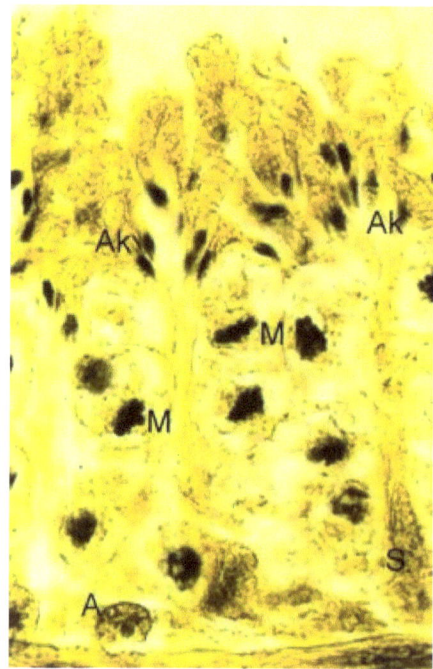

VI Cytokinesis Stage

Fig.8: Seminal epithelium, cat, xxxEH: cytokinesis stage with A-spermatogonia(A), sertoli cell (S), metaphasis spermatozytes (M), akrosomal spermatids (Ak).

Regulation
Leydig cells produce under hypothalamic control androgens with systemic and local effects. Between Leydig and Sertoli cells a chemical communication goes on to regulate the spermatogenesis (gonadocrinin, oxytocin, vasopressin, endorphine, testibumin, transferring, inhibin, antiakrosin).

Oogenesis
Oogenesis has a prenatal phase in the ovary of the female fetus, where the primordial germ cells divide to oogonia, which are forming together with a flat layer of follicle epithelium primordial follicles. They are mitotically active up to, and in carnivores and ruminants, even beyond parturition. Most of these several millions follicles will later degenerate to atretic follicles, only a selected smaller group enters the prophase of meiosis as primary oocytes in primary follicles. After entering the prophase of the first meiotic division there is a rest of the meiosis in the postnatal phase. Completion of the first meiotic division does not take place until the female reaches sexual maturity in the postpubertal phase. Then the folliculogenesis with the formation of tertiary follicles is a cyclic event and ovulation begins. Before or during ovulation secondary oocytes and the first polar bodies are released. The second maturation division is completed after fertilization, except in the dog and the horse, where both meiotic divisions occur after fertilization. In any case it is not possible to observe all steps of the meiosis in one slide of the ovary. In most of the ovarian follicles one can find only primary oocytes, which are arrested in a special diplotene stage of meiosis, called dictyotene, with partial reestablished euchromatin and a nucleolus in order to keep cell metabolism. In contrast to the male, the cytokinesis is also unequal. The oocyte keep most of the cytoplasm, the polar bodies contain only a minimum of it. A true ovum, as a female gamete with the haploid set, never exists, since the fertilized cell finishing the second meiotic division is already the zygote (2N).

Gametes
Gametes are among the most specialized cells in the organism. They are haploid cells with a male or female set of chromosomes.

Normal Chromosome sets (2N): Dog, chick 78, Horse 64, Donkey 62, Cattle, goat 60, Sheep 54, Men 46, Pig, cat 38

Drosophila type in mammals: AA (autosomes) XX (heterosomes) = female; AAXY = male
Abraxas type in birds: AAXX = male; AAXY = female
Protenor type in insects: AAXX = female; AAX = male

The male gametes have more or less the same principal structure in common, condensed chromosomes in the head, an acrosomal cap and a highly specialized, motile tail. They are called sperm cells or spermatozoa. The female gamete is the fertilized egg cell after the division of the second polar body only for a very short time. The ovulated preova are primary or secondary oocytes. Together with their sheaths, which are the zona pellucida, the corona radiata and eventual secondary sheaths like shells (birds) or neozonae (mammals), they are called eggs. In contrast to the uniform spermatozoa, the female eggs are classified dependent on the amount and the distribution of yolk (deuteroplasm) stored in the cell. Birds have macrolecithal (poly-, telolecithal), amphibians have mesolecithial (anisolecithal), and placental mammals have microlecithal (oligolecithal, isolecithal) eggs. This depends on inner or outer development (inner or outer insemination) giving the cells different sizes.

Average egg cell sizes (mm): Mouse 0.09, Cat 0.13, pig and Dog 0.14, Horse 0.14, Ruminants 0.15, Trout 1.0, Frog 1.5, Chicken 25

Oestrous cycle

To make a pregnancy possible all female mammals undergo cyclic changes of the behaviour and the morphology of the reproductive organs stimulated by hormones, light and temperature. Mammals with an oestrus once a year are monoestrous, others are dioestrous or polyoestrous, that is, they show oestrous behaviour at regular intervals throughout the year. Cats are polyoestrous, but have two breeding seasons a year; the cycle is without ovulation or has a provoked ovulation. The cycle has different phases called prooestrous, oestrous, postoestrous and between two oetrous phases the dioestrous or interoestrous phase. The duration of oestrous is different: mouse and rat 4-6 days (with 3-24 hours of oestrous), pig d21 (d2-3), horse d21-22 (d4-6), cattle d21 (12-24h), sheep d16-17 (d1), goat d20-21 (d1), cat anovulatory (no ovulation) d14-21 (d8), cat with ovulation d30-75 (d4-6), dog 6 months (d14-21).

Ovarian cycle

In cortex of the mature ovary primordial follicles are activated to grow to primary follicles with cubic follicle epithelium. Secundary follicles show a bigger egg cell, surrounded by a zona and 2-3 layers of follicle epithelium. Tertiary follicles have a cavity with fluid. During oestrous one or more of these become huge Graafian follicles and are ovulated.

In the postoestrous phase from the remnants of these follicles the corpus luteum is formed. Developmental abnormalities are common as persistent follicles and corpora lutea, cysts or anostrous, animals wihich are normally unfertil.

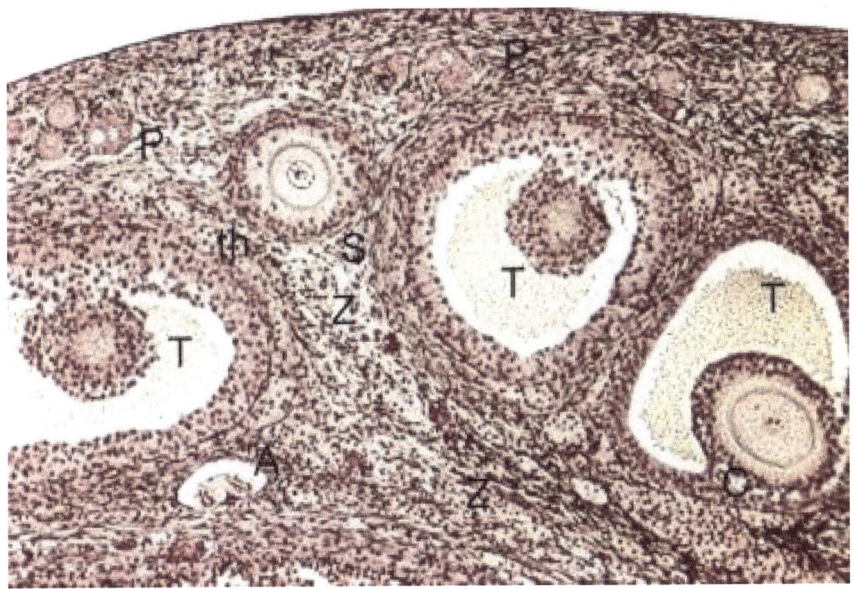

Fig.9: Ovary, cat, xxHE: primary follicles (P), secondary follicles with bigger oocytes and zona pellucida (S), tertiary follicles with an antrum (T), cumulus (C) and theca (th), intermediate cells (Z), atretic follicles (A).

Uterine cycle

In the prooestrous phase endometrial proliferation is significant. In cats and dogs also bleeding occurs. In the postoestrous phase the secretion of the endometrial glands is leading to the mucous phase of oestrous in cats. In the dioestrous phase the endometrium is reduced, what is causing the menstruation in primates.

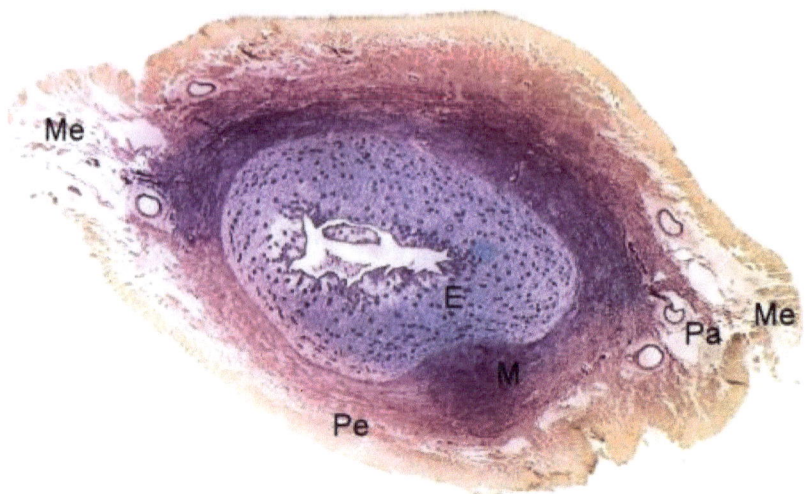

Fig.10: Uterus, dog, dioestrous, xHE: reduced endometrium (E), myometrium (M), perimetrium (Pe), parametrium with blood vessels (Pa) and mesometrium (Me).

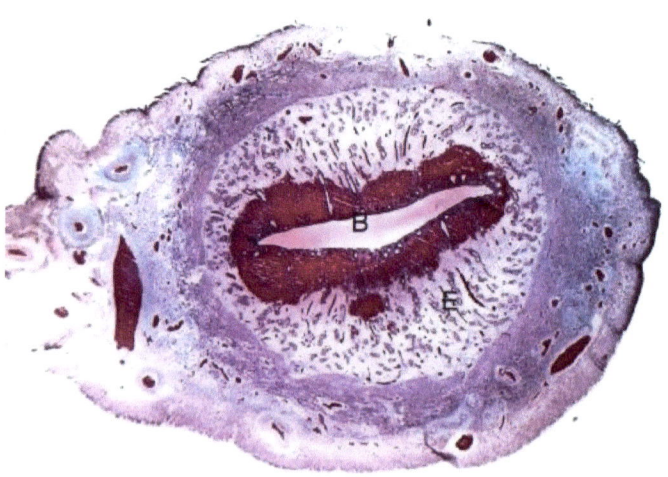

Fig.11: Uterus, dog, prooestrous, xHE: endometrium (E) with bleeding (B).

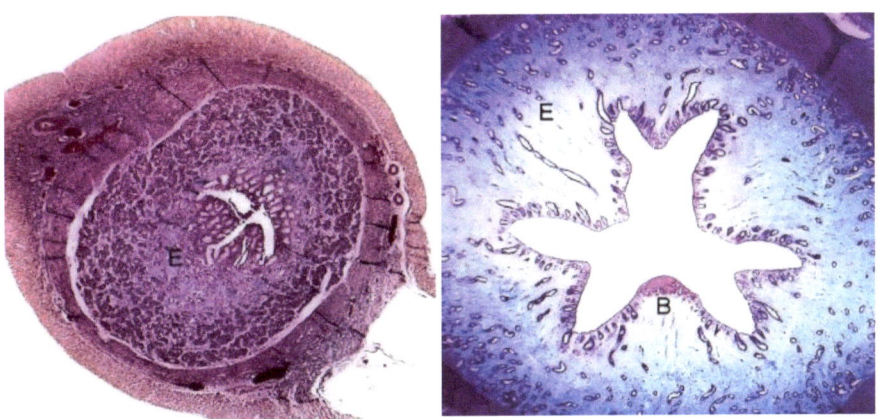

Fig.12 (let side): Endometrium, dog, oestrous, xGRA: endometrium with growing glands (E) and remnants of the bleeding (B). **Fig.13 (right side):** Uterus, dog, prostoestrous, xHE: endometrium with proliferated glands (E).

Vaginal cycle

In many species, especially mouse and rat, the vaginal epithelium shows also cyclic changes. Normally some epithelial cells and rounded cells (mainly lymphocytes) are found in vaginal smears. During oestrous the epithelium is characterized by a marked cornification (keratinization); during postoestrous many rounded cells are present.

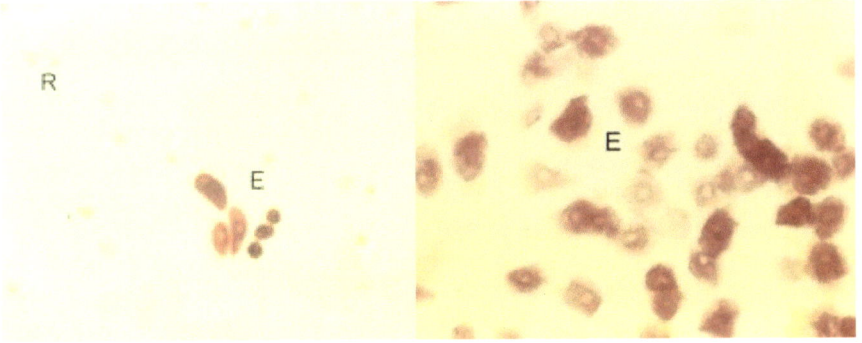

Fig.14 (left side): Vaginal smear, mouse, dioestrous, xxxPAP (Papaniculou stain): rounded cells (R) and epithelium (E). **Fig.15 (right side):** Vaginal smear, mouse, oestrous, xxxPAP: cornification of the epithelium (E).

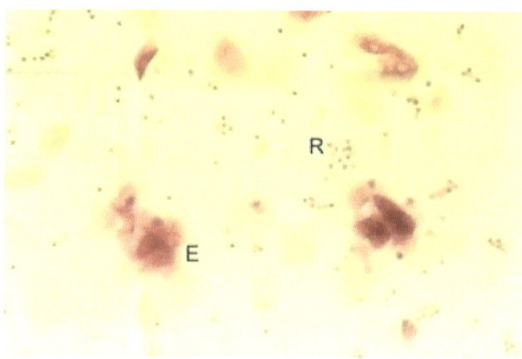

Fig.16: Vaginal smear, mouse, postoestrous, xxx PAP: many rounded cells (R) and epithelium (E).

Fertilization

Fertilization is the fusion of the male and female gametes to initiate the development of a new individual. It is preceded by the release of the oocyte (ovulation) and spermatozoa (ejaculation), and their unification in the female genital tract (insemination), naturally performed during mating (coitus) or by means of artificial insemination. Today it is also possible to unite both in vitro. The release of gametes, mating and insemination is normally a cyclic event, connected to changes in structure and function of the genital organs, regulated by many internal and external factors, which are subject of specialized veterinary scientific fields like animal reproduction, theriogenology, artificial insemination and gene manipulation. Embryology is more focusing to the following events started by fertilization leading to a new individual.

Ovulation is the rupture of one or more Graafian ovarian follicles. It can be spontaneous or induced (cat, rabbit). The ruptured follicle is transformed into a copus luteum, an important endocrine structure; its secretions produce uterine changes facilitating the implantation and maintenance of the pregnancy. The oocyte is flushed into the uterine tube, where normally the fertilization takes place between 12-24 hours after ovulation. Sperm cells are transported by muscular contractions to the uterine tube. They remain viable for several days (6-7 days in carnivores, horses, up to 70 days in turkeys) after their capacitation, but the oocyte viablility is only about 24 hours. The **capacitation** process (5-6 houres) involves the removal of glycoprotein coats and the activation of acrosomal enzymes in the spermatozoa. Fertilization can be subdivided into three main phases: Impregnation, Reduplication and Conjugation.

Impregnation

The impregnation starts with the penetration of the barriers between the female germ cell and the spermatozoon: the corona radiata (may have disappeared already), the zona pellucida and the oocytolemm. It is thought that these to be overcome by the action of the acrosomal enzymes of the sperm. Receptor mediated processes lead to a dropping potential of the egg cell, an increase of intracellular calcium and the release of cortical vesicles after the penetration of the first sperm cell. These cortical vesicles are creating (enzymatic) the fertilization membrane and a perivitelline space between oocytolemm and zona, to prevent additional sperm cells from fusing with the egg cells to block polyspermy. This is due to a chemical change of the zona (zona reaction). The 2nd meiotic division of the oocyte is completed producing the ovum and the 2nd polar body. The presence of the 2nd polar body is therefore, a sure evidence of fertilisation. Meanwhile the sperm cell head is fusing with the membrane and a conception hillock. The sperm is then enclosed completely or partially (in some domestic species only the head) into the egg cell, stimulating its development.

Reduplication
After a short rest the ovum and the enclosed sperm cell head are reconstructing their chromosomes, reduplicate them, and establish a male and a female pronucleus and a spindle apparatus. The sperm cell delivers the centriols for the first division.

Conjugation
Both pronulei move towards each other, fusing their chromatids and form in this way the tetraploid zygote. After a second rest of different duration, it is dividing, producing the first two blastomeres of the new individual. This happens about 60-68 hours post coitum in the cat.

Results of fertilization
1. It is the end of the meiosis and the initiation of cleavage, 2. It is the amphimixis with the restoration of the diploid chromosomal set, 3. It is the determination of the genetic sex.

Abnormalities
1. Twinning in uniparous animals
a. dizygous, when two separate ova are fertilized.
b. monozygous, when one ovum is fertilized but subsequently divided.

2. Polyspermy
Occasionally more than one spermatozoon penetrates the egg and several pronulei occur (common in the pig). Normally these polyploid zygotes die at a very early stage of development. Polyspermy is physiological in birds and produces merocytotic nuclei.

3. Parthenogenesis and Merogony
-is partial development without fertilization, physiological in avertebrates.

4. Superfecundation
-is the successive fertilization of two or more eggs by two or more different males (common in carnivores).

5. Superfetation
-is the fertilization of eggs in an already pregnant female (common in pigs and cattle).

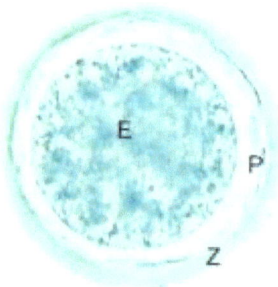

Fig.17: Fertilized egg cell of the cat, xxx, unstained: egg cell with yolk platelets (E), perivitelline space (P), transformed zona (Z).

Early Development

The early development starts with the onset of cell divisions, called cleavage, because furrows due to the divisions can be seen from outside. The zona is still intact at that time, the cells getting smaller and smaller, forming blastomeres, therefore the process is also called blastogenesis, and the whole structure blastomerula. The pattern of cleavage depends upon the egg cells type (yolk content), and is regulated by the cortical plasma. In poultry (birds, monotremata) it is a partial cleavage, because of the high yolk content. In mesolecithal eggs (amphibians) it is total, but inequal, and in our domestic mammals, where the egg contains only a small amount of yolk in form of scattered yolk platelets, it is a total, equal cleavage (amphioxus, marsupialia, eutheria). The first group has therefore a meroblastic type, the other groups have a holoblastic type of cleavage, where the first division occur at the long axis of the cytoplasm and the subsequent division tends to be at the right angle to the previous one. After some divisions, cleavage in mammals is getting asynchronous. The results is a cell mass of about 19-31 cells, resembling a small mulberry, termed morula, formed by morulation. In cats the morula is found in the oviduct between 72-124 hours after conception, its corona is already disintegrated, but its zona is still intact. At this stage the HY-antigen (male embryos) is already expressed.

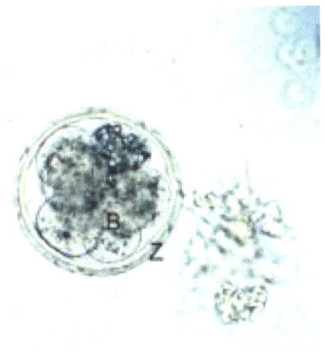

Fig.18: Blastumerula, sheep, 7 cell stage, xxx, unstained: blastomere (B), zona (Z).

During the first week of gestation the blastomeres lose their spherical appearance, being tightly packed inside the zona, which is oval, expanded but still intact. Intercellular fluid starts to appear and coalesce into a cavity, the blastocoele. The enlarged conceptus is now termed blastocyst in the blastulation period. Its cells are not indentical. An inner mass of cells forms the dorsal embryoblast or embryonic disk, and outer cells are forming the trophoblast. In general it can be said that the embryoblast gives rise to the embryo proper and the trophoblast cells facilitate the absorption of nutrients early in development and later participate in the development of the extraembryonic membranes and placenta. The zona disappears between the 1st and the 2nd week of development. This is the hatching of the blastocyst.

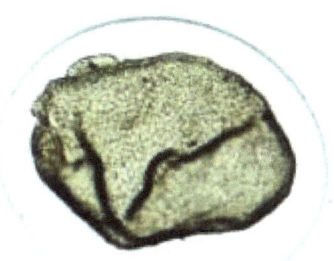

Fig.19: Blastocyst with zona, cat, 8 days, xxx, unstained.

Amphibians have no separated embryoblast and trophoblast, but there is a difference between the dorsal micromeres and the yolk-rich macromeres, which will give later raise to the endodermal cells. In birds with a meroblastic cleavage, the subgerminal cavity separates the central embryonic disc (blastoderm) and marginal syncytial trophoblast from the underlying yolk. In order to understand the gastrulation of mammals it is necessary to know these two extremes. The holoblastic amphibians, the meroblastic birds and as an intermediate type the mammals, which are holoblastic, but show similarities to the meroblastic type, by developing an embryonic disc. It is because eutherian mammals got secondary oligolecithal eggs, due to the prolonged, placental development, while protherian mammals have still polylecithal eggs. The meaning of blastulation is to enable the formation of the three germ layers during gastrulation.

Because mammalian morulae or blastocysts are preimplantation stages, they can be taken from a donor female into a buffered tissue culture medium, may be stored frozen in liquid nitrogen for a longer period to be transferred to another female. This technique of embryo transfer has nowadays a widespread commercial application. Embryo transfer may be coupled with invitro-fertilization, cloning and gene transfer.

Morphogenesis

Gastrulation starts during the 2nd week in most domestic mammals as the formation of the three germ layers, what is important for the inductive interaction of overlaying layers to form primitive organs and make the formation of a body form possible. This interaction is the effect of different genes, continuously regulating the further differentiation and determining the prospective potency of certain cells to their actual expression. The process is started very early in so-called mosaic eggs, later in so-called regulation eggs. Misinterpretation of experiments on different egg types lead to the former theories of preformation and epigenesis. Up to the 18th century followers of the preformation theory believed that the egg or the sperm cell contained a preformed small new individual, which only needs to grow, whereas the followers of the epigenesis theory believed in a complete regulation. The type of gastrulation like blastulation depends on the yolk content of the egg cell. The mesolecithal amphibian blastula invaginate the outside cells to form all germ layers. In contrast to that, domestic mammals (secondary oligolecithal) like meroblastic birds form the endoderm by delamination from the outer ectoblast, but the mesoderm by invagination between ecto- and entoblast, forming the primitive streak, what also establishes the embryonic axis. The cranial end of the streak is the enlarged primitive node (Hensen's node), from which the head process forms the cranially growing notochord and laterally spreading cells are forming the

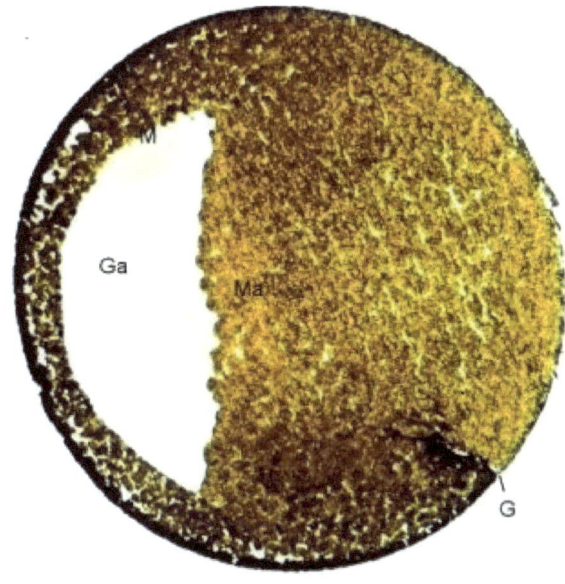

Fig.20: Gastrula, frog, xx, picroblue: gastroporus (G), gastrocoel (Ga), mircromeres (M), macromeres (Ma).

mesodermal plate. Only two circular zones are not invaded by the mesoderm, the prechordal plate (later buccopharyngeal membrane) in front of the notochord and the cloacal membrane behind the primitive streak, and remain, therefore as a bilaminar structure. The mesoderm continues to spread peripherally beyond the limits of the embryonic disc and gives rise to the extraembryonic mesoderm. These events are on principle the same in all vertebrates however in detail there are many differences. In domestic mammals we can find four main types and several subtypes of early development.

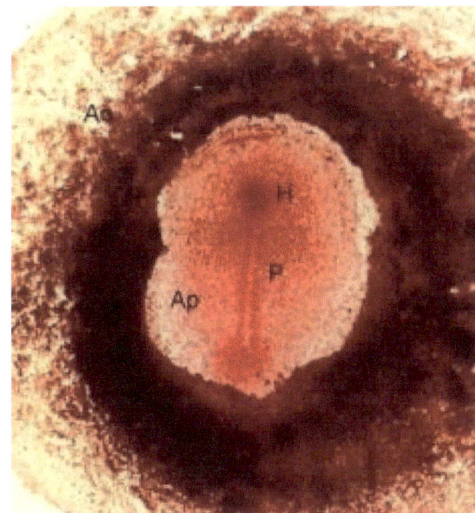

Fig.21: Blastoderm, chick, total, 10 hours, x, carmalaun: Area pellucida (Ap), Area opaca (Ao), Hensens node (H), primitive streak (P).

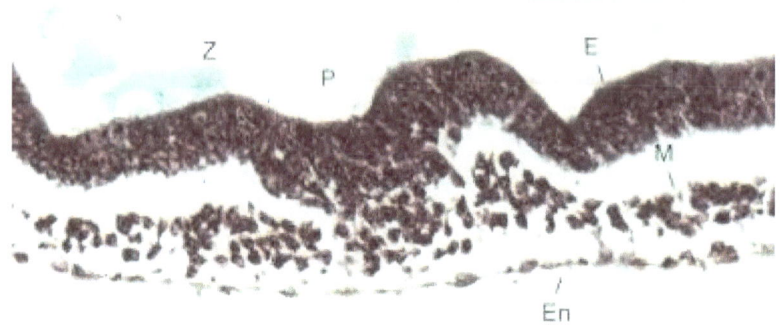

Fig.22: Gastrula, cat, 12 days, transversal, xxHE: ectoderm (E), entoderm (En), mesoderm (M), primitive streak (P), endometrial fluid (Z).

Neurulation

Neurulation is a series of folding during the 3rd week to form primitive organs and to establish the primitive body form from the flat embryonic disc. The neural plate invaginates to a neural groove, flanked by the neural folds (Periodus sulci neuralis initialis of the neurula) induced by the notochord. Also the mesoderm undergoes a rapid proliferation and becomes subdivided into different parts (Periodus mesodermalis et mesenchymalis of the coelomatula):

    a. the axial mesoderm (notochord)
    b. the paraxial mesoderm (somites)
    c. the intermediate mesoderm (somite stalk)
    d. and the lateral plate mesoderm

The paraxial mesoderm around the notochord is condensing and starts to develop in a cranio-caudal sequence primitive segments in form of paired somites (Periodus sulci neuralis maturi et somitorum immaturorum of the metamerula). These are still connected to the lateral plate in form of short stalks, the intermediate mesoderm. The lateral plate is separated into an inner splanchnic (visceropleura) lining the entodermal primitive gut and yolk sac and an outer somatic (somatopleura) mesoderm lamella. The cavity in between is the coelom, which will later form the body cavities. Both lateral plate and the coelom have an embryonic and an extraembryonic part. The visceropleura soon develops the first blood vessels. These elevate, converge and fuse in the dorsal midline, forming the neural tube with a cranial and caudal neuropore. The fusing ectodermal ridges on both sides are the neural crests. Notochord, neural tube, neural crests, somites and yolk sac are primitive organs, transitory structures, forming later parts of different permanent organs. The neural tube elongates rostrally, forming brain vesicles inside the head process, which overgrows the cardial and pericardial anlagen in front of the prechordal plate. Otic, optic, olfactory and hypophyseal placodes are distict at the head.

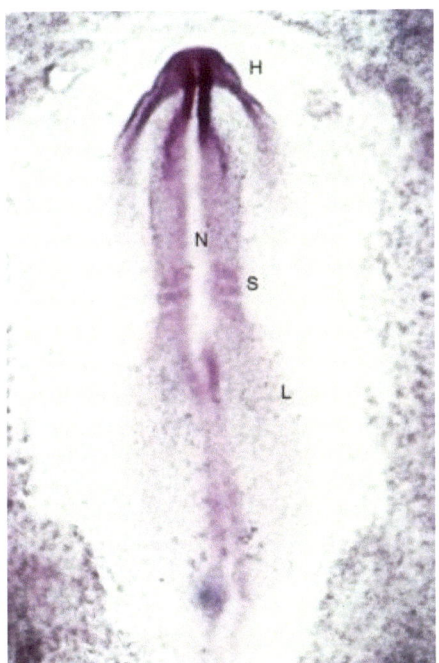

Fig.23: Chicken, total, 20 hours, xCarmalaun: head process (H), lateral plate (L), neural groove (N), somites (S).

Fig.24 (below): Chicken, transversal, 36 hours, xxHE: primitive aorta connected to early vessels (A), notochord (C), coelom (Coe), ectoderm (Ec), entoderm (En), notochord (N), somites (S), somatopleura (Sp), visceropleura (Spl).

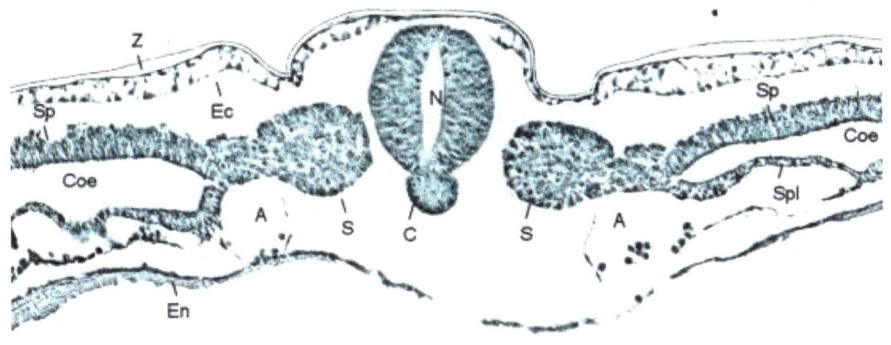

After this initial elevation of the head, craniocaudal and also lateral body folds are formed to separate the embryo with head, body and tail from the now underlying extraembryonic tissues, which are connected by the umbilical stalk to the body. The prechordal plate and pericard is reflected under the head, transformed to the heart bulge and the buccopharyngeal membrane at the bottom of the primitive mouth sinus. The heart tube is reflected, forming a mesodermal fold, called septum transversum.

Inside the embryo by this process the gut is transformed to a tube with a fore-, mid- and hindgut. The rostral foregut expands beneath the head process as the primitive pharynx. The openings to the umbilical stalk are the cranial and caudal intestinal portals. The hindgut with the outgrowing allantoic diverticulum is closed by the cloacal membrane. The gut communicates with the vasculated yolk sac at first widely and later by the narrow vitellointestinal duct. After the body form is established a convenient way of estimating the stage of development is to measure the length of the embryo from the crown to the rump. This crown-rump length can be used to estimate actual age by reference to conversion tables.

Embryonal development

During the embryonal period not only the placenta is formed, but also primitive organs are transformed and all permanent organs are developed in the beginning of the organogenesis. The embryonal period is subdivided by the main events to 6 further periods (periodus tubi neuralis, periodus pharyngealis initialis, periodus pharyngealis ultima, periodus gemmarum membrorum initialis, periodus gemmarum membrorum sera, periodus labii fissi with the stages 9-16 in the domestic cat, the first half of the pregnancy), in which the neural tube, the primitive pharynx, and the limb buds become visible.

Extraembryonic Membranes and Implantation

The free blastocyst is nourished by endometrial secretions. This is not sufficient anymore for the growing embryo. Therefore simultaneously with the process of body folding, a system of extraembryonic membranes is established in all land living vertebrates during the 2nd and 3rd week of development. These begin to make contact to the uterine mucosa during the process of implantation. The embryo becomes attached to the uterus, thus establishing a close link between embryonal and maternal tissue necessary for the development of a placenta, the definitive organ for nutrition of the fetus. The Implantation of most of the domestic mammals like horse, ruminants, carnivores and pig is central in the lumen of the uterus, excentric, antimesometrial in the mouse, rat, squirrel, and interstitial (inside the mucosa) in man, bats and guinea pigs. The time of the implantation is different: sow 10-12 days (112-115 days of gestation), Ewe 10-15 (144-152), Queen 13-14 (63-65), Cow 16-18 (279-285), Bitch 17-18 (58-65), Mare 35-42 (329-345).

Implantation is regulated by many factors and is connected to structural and physiological changes in the endometrium. The endometrium prepares the implantation by growing in thickness, and moves also the blastocyts to distribute them along both horns. Intra- and transuterine migration may occur as a result. In rare cases ectopic implantation can be the result of disturbances of the complex mechanism, when a fertilised ovum is lost into the peritoneal cavity and becomes implanted there. Wild animals can have retarded implantation.

Yolk Sac

The yolk sac is formed when endoderm spreads around the inner surface of the trophoblast forming the bilaminar omphalopleure. In birds it actually contains a mass of yolk, though in mammals it does not. However it continues to form in a similar manner but performs rather different functions. The extraembryonic mesoderm spreads outwards, progressively separating the yolk sac from the trophoblast by the formation of an extraembryonic coelom. Only the most distal part of the yolk sac stays in contact to the trophoblast and develops a temporary choriovitelline placenta in carnivores and the horse. Blood vessels develop within the wall, rich also of hemopoietic tissue and form the vitelline vessels. Because of inverted germ layers, laboratory mammals have the yolk sac also as an extraembryonic membrane.

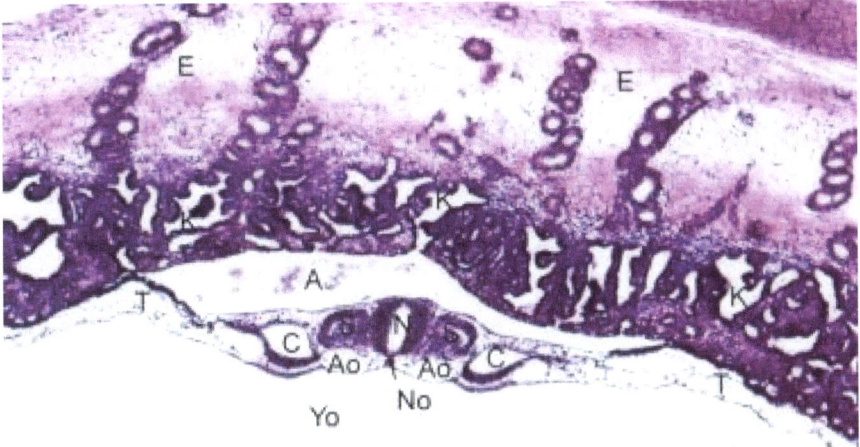

Fig.25: Embryo, cat 14d, xxHE: amnion cavity (A), paired aortae (Ao), coelom (C), endometrium with coiled glands (E), the mouth of the glands are forming krypts (K), neural tube (N), notochord (No), extraembyronic membranes attached to the emdometrium (T), lumen of the yolk sac (Yo).

Chorion
The chorion develops from the trophoblast, when the mesoderm separates it together with the extraembryonic coelom from the yolk sac. The chorion becomes a very large sac, especially in the pig and the ruminants. The secondary chorion fuses with other membranes, starts to produce villi on the surface and get vascularized by chorioallantoic vessels.

Amnion
In some species the trophoblast is folding and overgrowing the embryonic disc and finally fuses to form the amnion. This completes not only the amnion, but also the chorion. In other species the amnion is formed by cavitation in the trophoblast material overlying the embryonic disc. Accumulation of fluid causes the amnion to become a large sac, getting into contact with other extraembryonic membranes and forming the amnio-chorion in ruminant and pigs and the allantoamnion in carnivores and the horse.

Allantois
The allantois is outgrowing from the hindgut into the extraembryonic coelom. Meanwhile the yolk sac regresses in size, the allantois enlarges greatly due to the accumulation of embryonal urine. Eventually the allantois fuses with the chorion and the amnion, and form by this the allantochorion and allantoamnion. The vessels associated with the allantois are the umbilical vessels, which are important in providing the embryonal vascular component of the placenta. The allantois of primates remains a vestigial structure and does not collect embryonal urine.

Placentation
After implantation a close relationship between the embryonal and the maternal circulatory system is established in a combined organ, the placenta, to make the embryonal nutrition, respiration and excretion possible. The embryonal parts are formed by the chorion; the maternal components are specialisations of the endometrium during the process of placentation. The primary chorion is avascular. First blood vessels are formed in the splanchnic mesoderm of the yolk sac, and later in the mesoderm of the allantois. Eventually, the avascular chorion fuses with the yolk sac or allantois and then becomes vascularized. Therefore the placental vessels are contained in the umbilical cord together with the vitellointestinal duct, the stalk of the allantois and loose embryonic connective tissue termed Wharton's jelly. The cord is lined on its outer surface by the amnion epithelium.

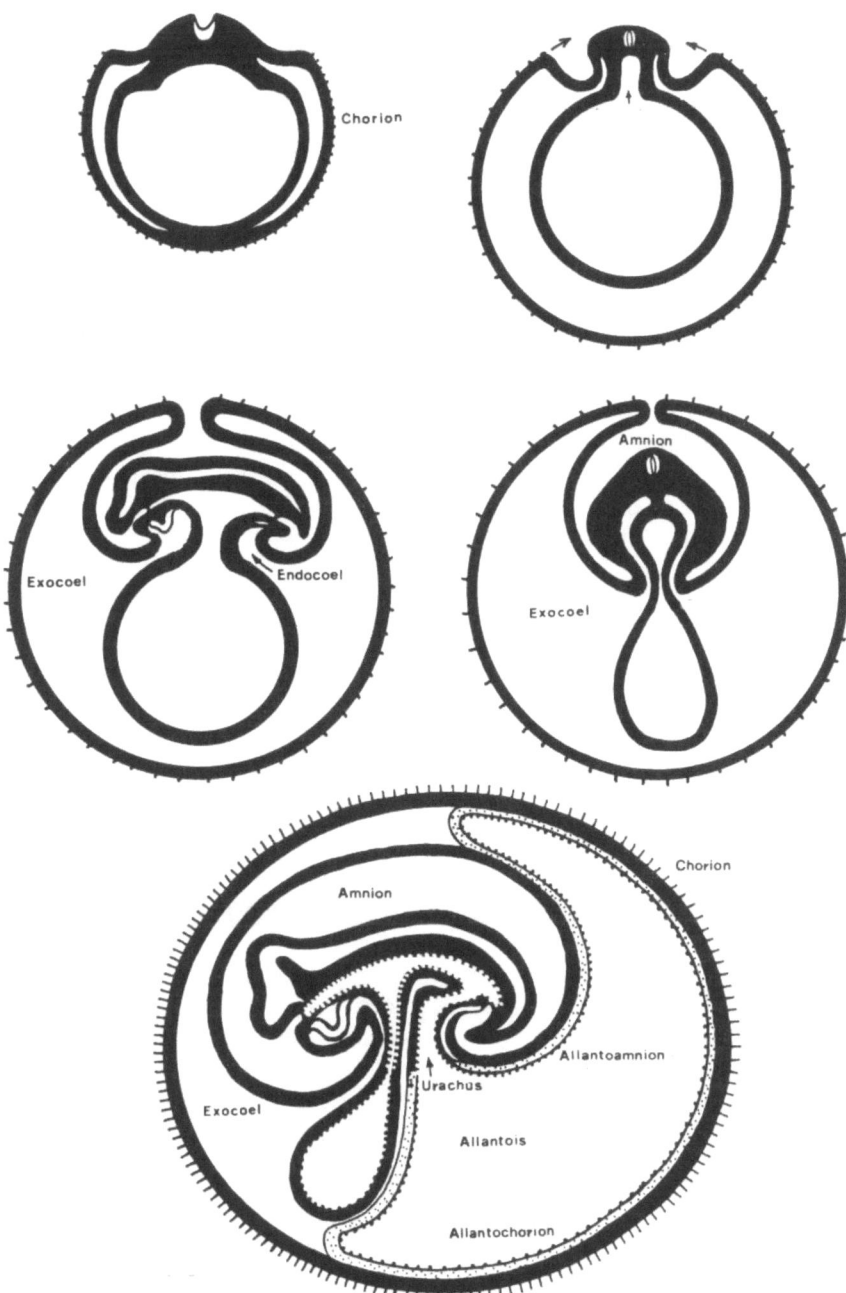

Fig.26: Development of the extraembryonic membranes (from Künzel and Knospe, 1987).

Classification of the placenta

Species differences are reflected in five main classification systems, based on different criteria as:

1. Extraembryonic membrane contribution

In horses and dogs in the first quarter of gestation a choriovitelline (omphaloid) placenta develops from the chorion and the attached yolk sac, later the yolk sac regresses and the chorioallantoic placenta develops.

2. Gross structure of the placenta

The secondary chorion has a smooth part (chorion leave) and a specialized part (chorion frondosum) with different surface projections. In the diffuse placenta (sow, mare) most of the chorionic sac is equipped with small villi. In the cotyledonary placenta (multiplex) the chorionic villi form tufts, cotyledons, which are attached to the endometrial prominences, caruncles. Together they form the 60-120 placentomes (ruminants). In the zonary placenta the frondose chorion forms a girdle (cranivores), and in the discoid placenta it forms a disc-shaped area (primates, rodents).

3. Architecture of the placenta

The three-dimensional structure of the interface between the maternal and embryonal tissues can be different. In the folded placenta it is in form of macroscopic folds or microscopic ridges (mare, sow), or in lamellae (carnivores). In the villous placenta, there are villi, fitting to maternal crypts, and in the labyrinthine placenta there is an intercommunicating network of villi and maternal blood vessels (carnivores, rabbit).

4. Type of interconnection

Depending on the degree of maternal-embryonal interconnection the endometrium is changed and the chorion anchored. In the nondeciduate placenta both components can be separated without much loss of endometrium, whereas in the deciduate placenta a functional part of the endometrium, the decidua, is shedded during parturition.

5. Fine structure of placenta

Embryonal and maternal vessels are more or less separated by different histological strutures, forming the placental barrier. In the epitheliochorial placenta these are the embryonal endothelium, mesenchyme, and chorion epithelium, the endometrial epithelium, connective tissue and the maternal endothelium (sow, mare and cow). If the endometrial epithelium is displaced, it is the syndesmochorial placenta (goat, sheep). In the endotheliochorial placenta the chorion reaches direct to the maternal endothelium (cranivores), and in the hemochorial placenta (primates, rodents) all three maternal layers are absent. If all layers are present the embryotrophe, which nourishes the embryo is fluid (histiotrophe), resorpted by the chorionic epithelium. If all maternal layers are absent the maternal blood is the nourishment (hemotrophe). In most of the species one can find different types in different locations (areolae, junctional zones, hematomes, and paraplacenta).

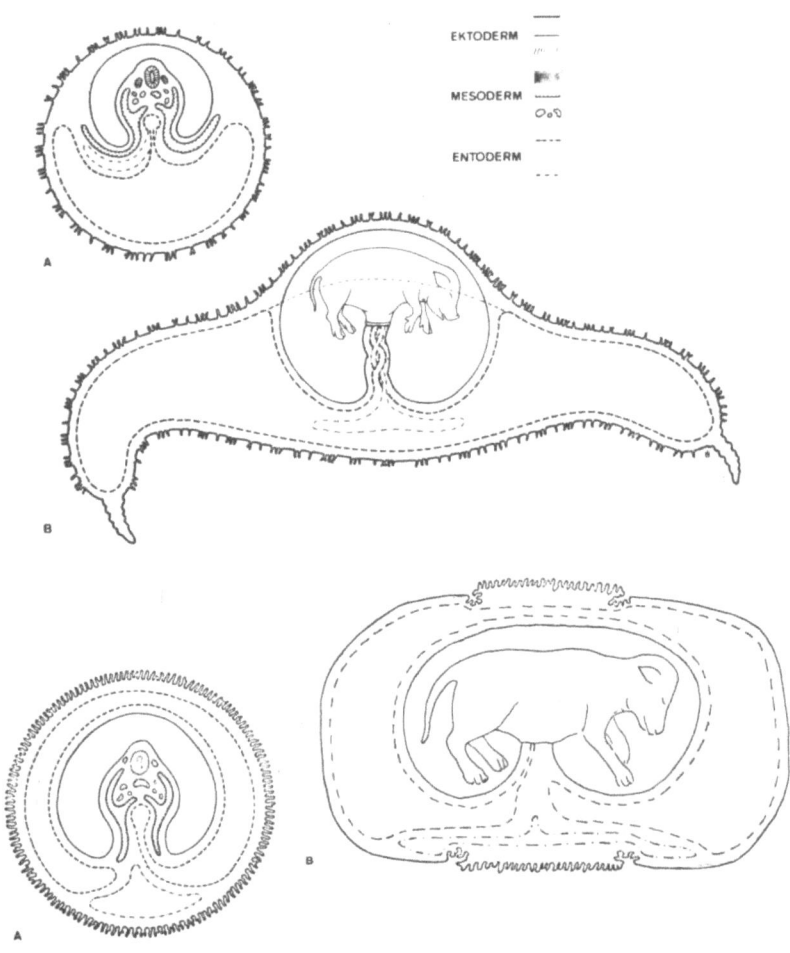

Fig.27: Extraembryonic membranes of the pig and dog (from Künzel and Knospe 1987).

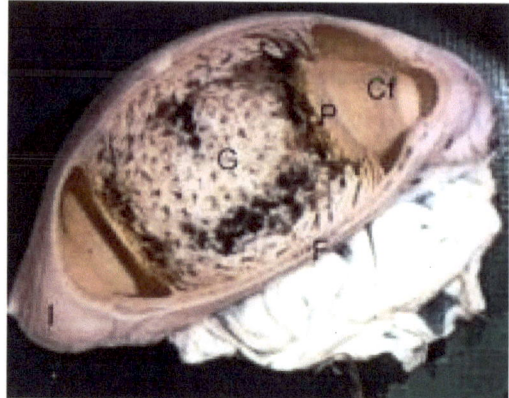

Fig.28: Placenta, cat, total: chorion leave (Cf), opened uterus forming a fruit chamber (F), placental girdle (G), internodium of the uterus (I), paraplacental region (P).

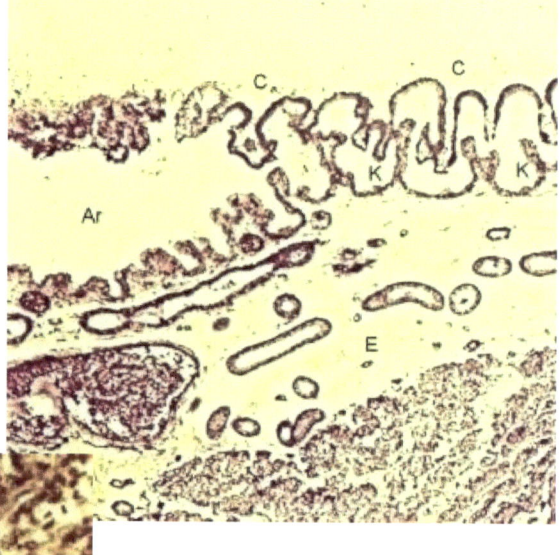

Fig.29: Placenta of the pig, xxHE: areolae (Ar), chorionic villi (C), endometrium (E) with krypts (K).

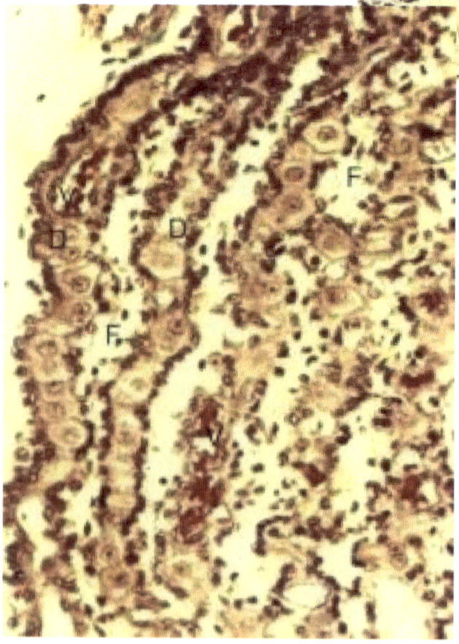

Fig.30: Placental labyrinth, cat, xxxHE: decidua cells next to maternal vessels (V), chorion vessels inside the embryonal lamellae (F).

The placenta is changing shape, size and structure during pregnancy. Many specialized trophoblast cells exist, like decidua cells, which are capable of phagocytosis, exchange and hormon production. In many species they produce chorionic gonadotropin (mares), placental lactogen (ruminants), estrogens, progesterones and other paracrine, metabolic factors. After birth the extraembryonic membranes and the placenta are forming the decidua. Malformations are avillous or diffuse placenta (ruminant).

The yolk sac placenta receives blood from the vitelline arteries, the oxygenated blood return through the vitelline vein. Left vitelline and right umbilical vein are reduced later on. In the chorioallantoic placenta there are the umbilical arteries and veins transporting the blood from and to the embryo via the umbilical cord. The umbilical cord measures 4-8 cm in carnivores, 25 cm in pigs, 10-25 cm in ruminants, and up to 60 cm in horses.

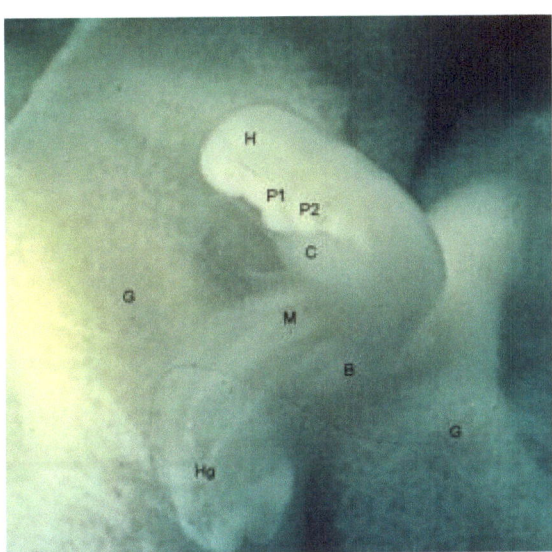

Fig.31: Tubula of the cat with 16 days, x, fixed but unstained: head with placodes and brain vesicles (H), the first two pharyngeal arches (P1, P2), heard inside the primitive pericard (C), open midgut (M), hindgut (Hg), shallow limb bud (B), girdle placenta (G).

Organogenesis

From the 3-4th week of gestation on in mammals different body parts and organs are formed by the germ layers and their primitive, transitory organs. This is a very complex process controlled by genes, different factors, hormones and inducers, simultaneously working in different organ systems. Therefore it is better to mention the different organ systems separately.

Fetogenesis and Histogenesis

With 28-32 days the fetal period starts (Periodus fetalis initialis). The early fetus grows rapidly and most organs have reached their definitive positions.

The forehead is prominent, eyes closed by the rapidly growing eyelids, short, triangular ear, tactile hair buds in the lips, typical mouth with mental cushion, the nose with keratinization at the planum, a short neck, the trunk relatively slim, the back with a slight lordosis, the heart and liver region are less protuberant and the hernia of the midgut ist withdrawn. The mammary buds are paramedial, the tail is free, all three major segments of the limbs are clearly demarcated, the fott is now pronated, the toes separated with pads and claws, but the genitals are still indifferent.

The late fetal period (Periodus fetalis definitiva), beginning with 44-48 days and ending with the birth, followed by the postnatal period, is mainly the period of further growth and histological differentiation of the organs and tissues - the so called histogenesis. Also these periods and their most important events are better mentioned together with the organ systems.

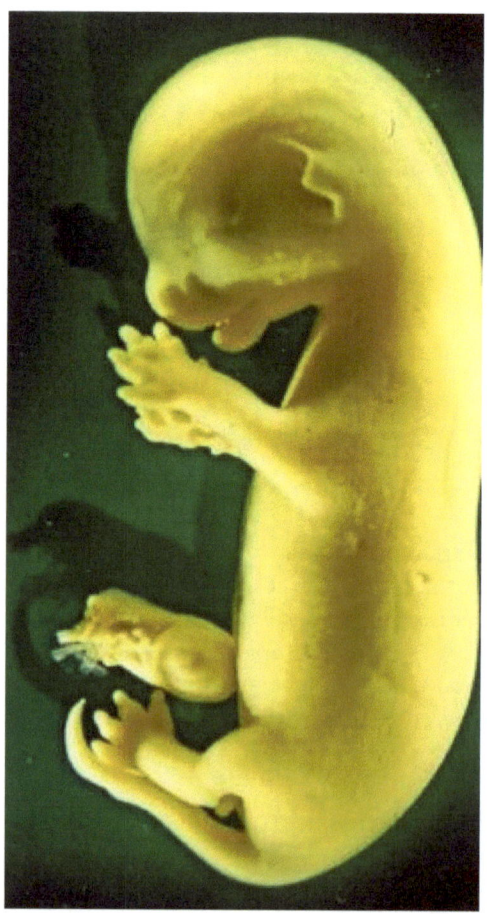

Fig.32: The early fetus of the cat (stage 18; 3.5 cm CRL).

The Cardiovascular System

Blood vessels
Heart, vessels and blood cells have the same origin in mesenchymal cells forming blood islets in the wall of the yolk sac. Outer cells flatten to form endothelial cells, inner cells transform to primitive hemocytoblasts as stem cells for blood cells, and intercellular fluid is the first plasma. First these vessels form a network later main stream vessels develop all over the embryo and extraembryonic membranes, linked up to the primitive heart.

Heart

Already in the second week mesoderm cells differentiate in front of the prechordal plate forming the cardiogenic area. During the third week the cardiogenic area is already transformed to the primitive heart with paired endocardial tubes, fusing later in the middle region, surrounded by the most cranial part of the coelom, the pericardial cavity.

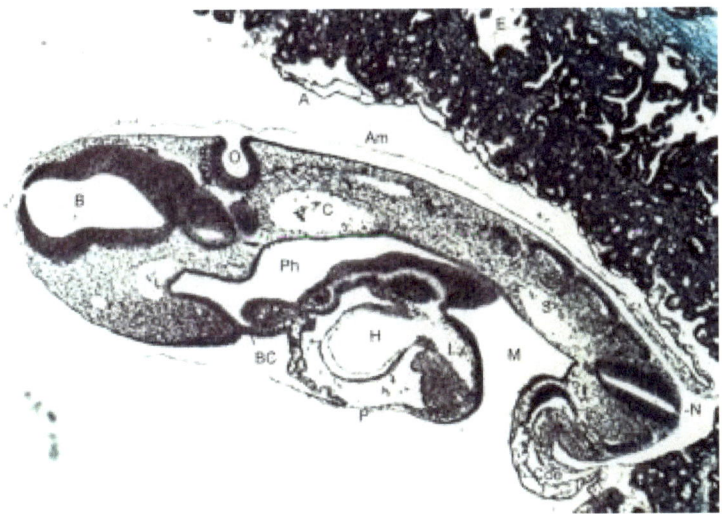

Fig.32: Cat embryo, 17 days, longitudinal section, xxtrichrome: allantochorion (A), amniochorion (Am), brain vesicle (B), cardinal vein (C), heart (H), pericardium (P), otic pit (O), primitive pharynx (Ph), branchial furrow (BC), midgut (M), neural tube (N), somites in transformation (S), somato- and visceropleura with the coelomic space (Coe).

The united heart tube has an inlet connected to the omphalomesenteric veins that drain the yolk sac and the cardinal veins that drain the embryonal body. The outlet supplies the paired primitive aortae and the omphalomesenteric arteries. During neurulation the heart is overgrown by the forming embryo and reflected ventrally to its head. This process is called the heart descend, reflecting the pericard ventrally and raises the inlet caudally and producing in this way the septum transversum.

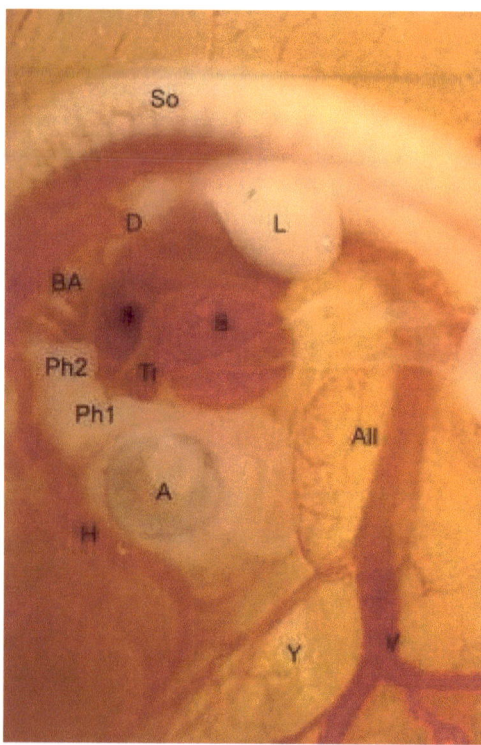

Fig.33: Chicken embryo, 5 days, xx unstained: head with cranial cardinal vein (H), optic cup (A), bulbus cordis (B), truncus (Tr), sinus venosus (S), duct of Cuvier (D), branchial arteries (BA), first and second pharyngeal arches (Ph1/2), limb bud (L), allantois vesicle (All), vitelline vein (V), yolk sac (Y).

Later paired umbilical veins from the chorioallantoic membranes are connected with the inlet of the heart. During the development of the pharyngeal arches, the ventral and dorsal primitive aortae are connected by several aortic arches, called branchial arteries. At the urogenital sinus umbilical arteries leave the aortae to the placenta. Inside the heart the lining endothelium forms the endocardium surrounded by the semi fluid cardiac jelly which later develops the myocardium. The cranial part will become the truncus arteriosus, bulbus and ventricles, the caudal part will form atria and sinus. Rapid growth forces the heart tube into a flexure with a ventro-caudal apex on the right side. This heart loop becomes subdivided because the atrial part enlarges to a transverse unpaired atrium that receives on both sides the sinus with the incoming cardinal, omphalomesenteric and umbilical veins. The subdivision between atrium and bulbus is marked by a constriction, the atrio-ventricular sulcus, between the ventricles and the truncus is the ventriculobulbic sulcus.

The left sinus is reduced after the obliteration of the left umbilical vein forming the coronary sinus. The right side forms the sinus venarum. The inner septation starts in the lumen of the atrium by a ridge, the primary septum, projecting to the lumen and forming the ostium primum. The definitive division between the two atria is achieved by a second septum left to the first.

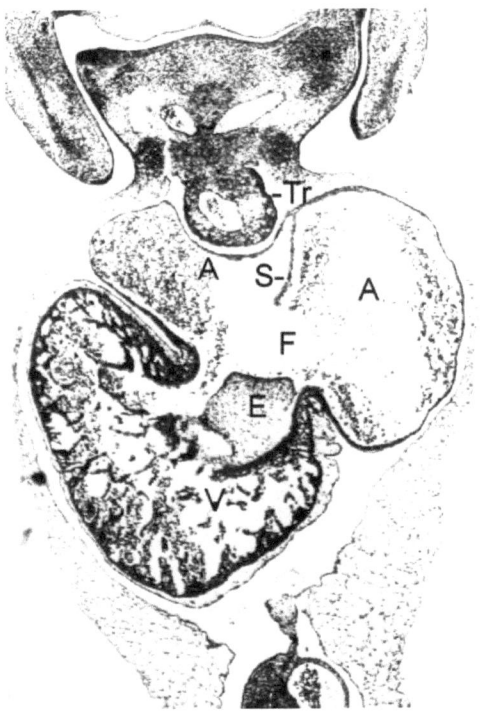

Fig.34: Chicken embryo, 5 days, horizontal section, xxHE: atria (A), endocardial cushion (E), primary ostium (F), primary septum (S), truncus (Tr), ventricle (V).

The free margin of this overlaps the ostium, forming the foramen ovale. The remnant of the primary septum forms a valve for it, which is closed after birth by the blood stream inversion (not in blue babies). Endocardial cushions divide the atrioventricular canal into a right and a left atrioventricular ostium.

The septation of the ventricle, bulb and truncus is achieved by the growth of two longitudinally endocardial ridges in the truncus. They fuse producing a partition. The interventricular septum appears as a falciform crest at the apex, extending and dividing the common cavity into right and left chambers. The two ventricles still communicate over the free edge, but are in separate communication with the atria through the paired slit-like opening of the atrioventricular canal. These are later forming the cusps of the valves.

The division of the ventricles is completed by fusion of the interventricular septum with the caudal cushion. The same process completes the division of the output, forming the aorta and the pulmonary trunk.

During further development of the atria the sinus venosus becomes incorporated into the right atrium. As result the cranial and caudal caval vein now open separately into the right atrium. A portion the primitive pulmonary vein becomes incorporated into the wall of the left atrium. Both atria later enlarge and develop the blind ending auricles. The development of valves is generated by localised mesenchymal thickenings around the margins of the AV orifices. At the free edges remaining tissue strands form the chordae tendinae. During the following histogenesis of the heart the coronary vessels and the conducting system is formed by differentiation from myocardial tissue. During the incorporation of the sinus venosus into the right atrium also the nodes develop. The heart commences almost as soon as muscle cells are formed, prior to the establishment of the conducting system, with beating.

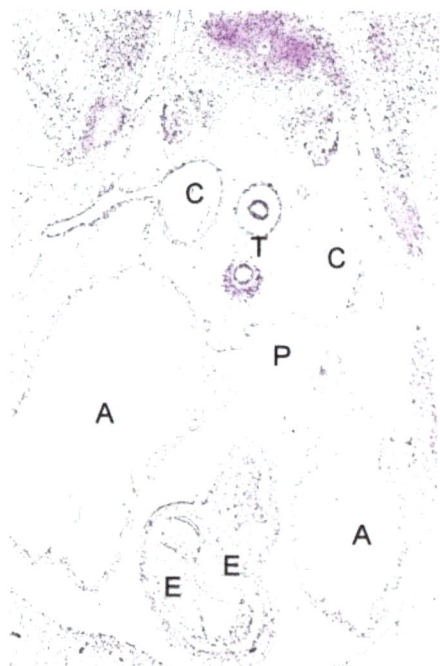

Fig.35: Cat embryo, 22 days, cross section, xxHE: atria (A), aortae (C), endocardial ridges (E), trachea and esophagus (T), primitive pericardial cavity (P).

It is not surprising that this complicated process can mishap leading to different heart malformations. Common in domestic mammals is the Acardie, Situs inversus, Ectopia cordis, where the heart is lacking or develops in an abnormal location. Common are also septal defects and the transposition of the great vessels, pulmonic stenosis (dog), subaortic stenosis (pig). Tetralogy of Fallot and the Eisenmenger syndrom are complex anomalies with ventricular and septal defects, over-riding aorta, right ventricular hypertrophy and pulmonic stenosis (not in Eisenmenger).

Arteries

From the truncus arteriosus six paired branchial arteries arise and run dorsally inside the pharyngeal arches and reach the dorsal aorta on either side. The dorsal aorta is paired in the early primitive form, later the right (left in birds) side is reduced. A number of branches arise in the abdominal region forming dorsal, lateral and ventral segmental arteries. The ventral unpaired omphalomesenteric artery develop in association with the developing gut. Lateral paired vessels are the urogenital and umbilical arteries. The umbilical arteries join the outgrowing allantoic sac, branches to the iliac arteries and run through the umbilical cord to the placenta.

The paired third branchial arteries are later transformed to the carotid arteries. The fourth forms the trunk of the subclavian artery on the right and the aortic arch on the left side. The arteries of the first, second and fifth are reduced and the arteries of the 6th arch form the pulmonary arteries. The left retains its connection to the dorsal aorta throughout fetal life as ductus arteriosus, which allows blood to pass from the pulmonary artery to the aorta. After birth this connection is lost, remnants are forming the ligamentum arteriosum. If the connection is not lost, a persistent ductus arteriosus is found. A persistent right aortic arch may form a ring around the trachea and the esophagus which leads to dysphagia.

Veins

Connected to the sinus is the duct of Cuvier on both sides with the cranial and caudal cardinal veins, the umbilical veins and the omphalomesenteric veins. The cardinal veins have subdivisions: the supracardinal vein in the head region and the subcardinal veins in the trunk.

By the development of the liver the omphalomesenteric veins form a network of hepatic veins: Vv. hepaticae advehentes to the liver and Vv. hepaticae revehentes to the heart. A shortcut between both is the venous duct (Ductus Arantii).

Again main stream tracts are developed and other branches reduced. The left cranial cardinal vein is joined by a new anastomotic branch to the right

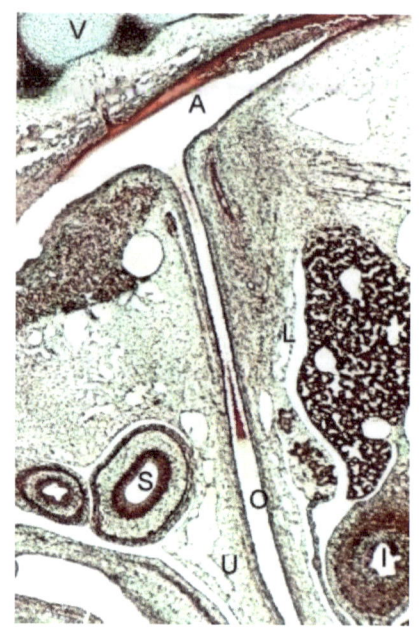

Fig.36: Cat embryo, 26 days, xxtrichrome: aorta (A), intestines (I), liver (L), A. omphalomesenterica (O), sinus urogenitalis with urachus (S), umbilical cord (U).

cranial cardinal vein, forming both internal jugular veins, the right cranial cardinal vein forms the terminal part of the cranial vena cava. The supracardinal veins form the azygos veins. The caudal vena cava has a complex development. Its terminal portion is derived from the right ompalomesenteric vein other parts are from subcardinal and hepatic (advehentes) veins. The distal portion of the right omphalomesenteric vein is forming the portal vein. The umbilical veins unite more or less caudal to the liver, where some blood is discharged into the hepatic sinusoids and much is passed directly to the caudal vena cava via the ductus venosus. Subcardial veins get in contact to inner organs, caudal body parts and cardinal veins.

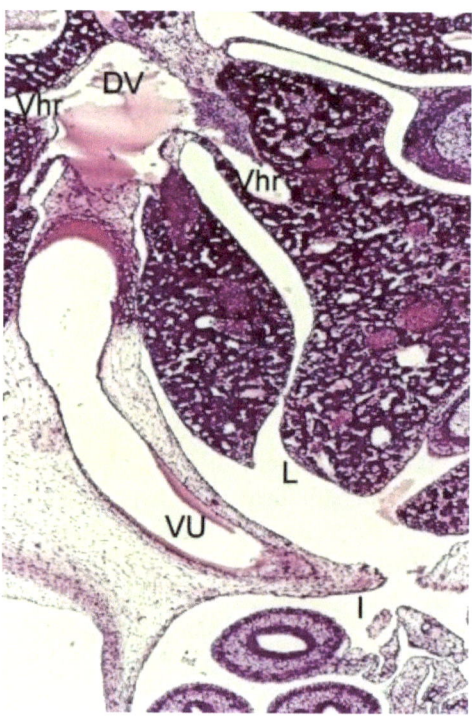

Fig.37: Cat embryo, 28 days, longitudinal section, xxHE: venous duct (DV), liver (L), intestines (I), hepatic revehent vein (Vhr), umbilical vein (VU).

Circulatory changes during birth

Oxygenated blood from the placenta is returned to the fetus by the umbilical veins within the umbilical cord. Over the venous duct, bypassing the liver it is brought to the caudal cava vein and mixes with the blood of the

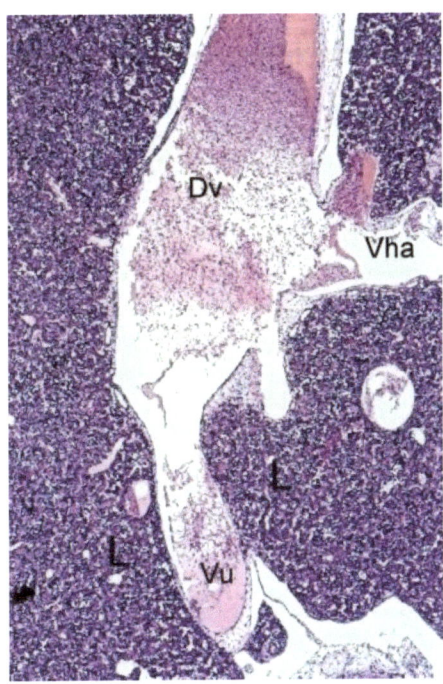

Fig.38: Cat embryo, 34 days, xxHE: venosus duct (Dv), liver with many blood islets (L), hepatic vein (Vha), umbilical vein (Vu).

hind part of the body. The blood then enters the right atrium and mixes with the blood of the head. A small part continues to the right ventricle and the pulmonary trunk, the larger part passes through the oval foramen to the left atrium, left ventricle and aorta. Parts of the right stream enter also the aorta via the arteriosus duct (Botalli). The mixed output of both ventricles supplies the body and leaves the embryo via the umbilical arteries. With birth and the interruption of the fetal circulation there is a decrease in oxygen, followed by initiation of pulmonary ventilation. The pressure in the right atrium is reduced, in the left atrium increased, what halts the shunt through the foramen ovale. Venosus and arteriosus ducts are closing over a period of several days.

Hematopoiesis

The hematopoiesis begins in the wall of the yolk sac. It is the megaloblastic period of hematopoiesis, where primitive blood cells are formed in small nests from mesenchymal cells. In a later period, the hepatolienal period, such hematopoietic clusters are found in some organs, especially the liver and spleen, and in the last third of gestation the bone marrow starts in the medullary period the hematopoiesis, like after parturition. Extramedullary hematopoiesis persists in the liver and spleen for a few weeks after birth and then gradually disappears.

Lymphatic System
Together with blood vessel also lymph vessel and larger lymphatic sacs are developed. In crossing points of this network, lymphnodes are developed as accumulations of differentiating mesenchymal cells. In the bone marrow and thymus (mentioned in chapter bone and primitive pharynx), the primary lymphatic organs, the lymphocytes develop from stem cells. Intense proliferation is accompanied by a selection of competent cells, which are then distributed throughout the body to all secondary lymphatic organs.

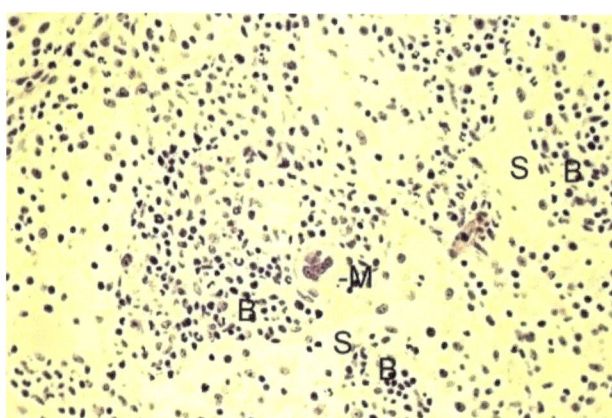

Fig.39: Lymphatic node of the cat, prenatal, xxxHE: hematopoietic spots (B) inside the mesenchyme with megakaryocytes (M) and blood sinus (S).

The spleen
The spleen develops in the dorsal mesogastrium, and is rotated together with the stomach (see there). The origin is the coelomic epithelium that proliferates into the underlying mesoderm. This blastema becomes vascularized, forming a reticular pattern, where also haematopoiesis starts. The white pulp develops later during the third trimester.

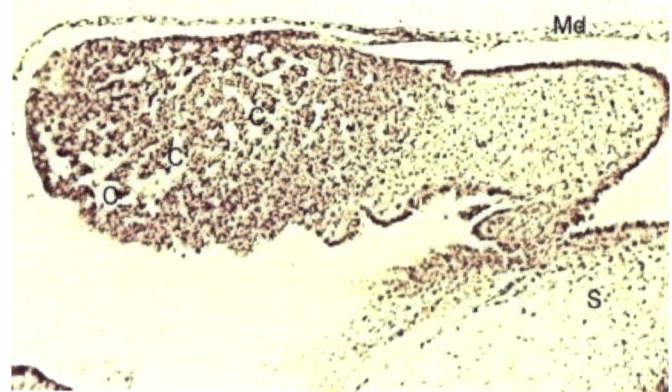

Fig.40: Chicken embryo 6 days, xxxHE: coelomic cell clusters in the early spleen (C), dorsal mesogastrium (Md), stomach wall (S).

The Digestive Apparatus

The digestive system originates from two sources: the ectodermal, primitive stomatodeum and the entodermal gut. Both are formed during neurulation and have contact to the lining mesenchyme. The gut is folded off the yolk sac and can be subdivided into three parts: foregut, midgut and hindgut. The foregut reaches from the buccopharyngeal membrane to the cranial intestinal portal with the primitive pharynx, stomach, lung, liver and pancreas as derivatives; the midgut from the cranial to caudal intestinal portal forming later the small intestines; and the hindgut from the caudal intestinal portal to the cloacal membrane developing large intestines and the urogenital sinus.

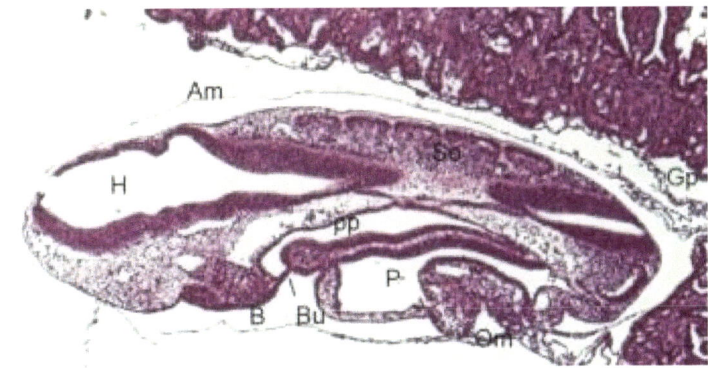

Fig.41: Cat embryo, 17 days, longitudinal section, xxHE: amnion (Am), maxillary process of the first pharyngeal arch (B), buccopharyngeal membrane (Bu), placental girdle (Gp), brain vesicles (H), liver and ompholomesenteric vein (Om), pericardial cavity (P), primitive pharynx (pp), somites (So).

Primitive Pharynx

The development of head and neck together with the face, the upper respiratory and the upper digestory system are connected with the development of the primitive pharynx and its transformation. With 14-18 days (cat) the pharyngeal arches are developing by the distribution of mesectodermal mesenchyme around the most cranial part of the gut, the primitive pharynx. With 18 days the buccopharyngeal membrane breaks down and the primitive pharynx is opened to the stomatodeum, which is surrounded by the first arch. The first arch soon develops an upper maxillary process and a lower mandibular process. The second arch (hyoid arch) is rapidly growing soon covering the third and fourth arch with the operculum. In this way the cervical sinus is formed. Arch 5 and 6 do not form surface elevations in mammals, but inside there are cartilage blastems, arch arteries, arch nerves and arch muscle blastems. Inside between the arches there are entodermal pharyngeal pouches, and outside between the arches there are ectodermal clefts. Pouches and clefts are connected without mesenchyme between, forming closing membranes. When the operculum is covering the caudal clefts, only the first cleft is visible from the outside.

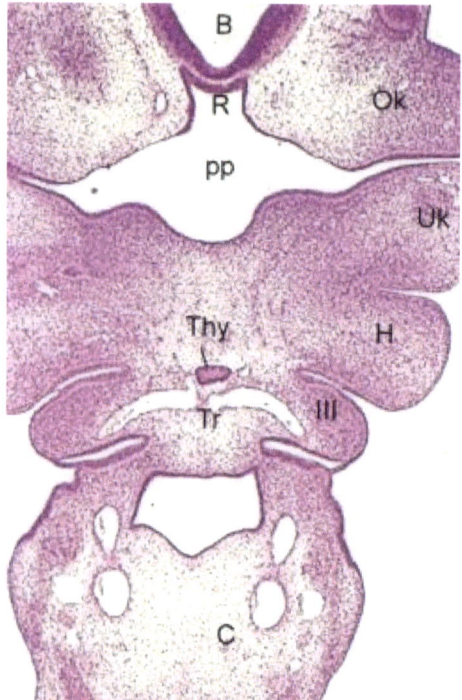

Fig.42: Sheep embryo, 15 mm, horizontal, xxHE: diencephalic vesicle (B), Rathke's pouch (R), maxillary process (Ok), mandibular process (Uk), hyoid arch (H), third arch (III), thyroid (thy), arterial trunk (Tr), cardinal veins (C).

Hypobranchial Region

The floor of the primitive pharynx is the hypobranchial plate. It is the source of the thyroid gland, parts of the tongue and the larynx. The rostral impar tubercle is forming together with lateral lingual swellings from the first pharyngeal arch the material of the distal 2/3 of the tongue. The hypobranchial eminence (copula) together with material from 2-4 arches are forming the proximal third of the tongue with connected muscles and glands. This is reflected in the complex innervation of the tongue by cranial nerve V, VII, IX, X, and XII, which are the nerves of the first, second, third, fourth arch and the nerve of the hypobranchial region. Between tuberculum impar and copula the thyroid placode is invaginated, first forming the thyroid vesicle, later the thyroid bulb, connected with the thyreoglossal duct to the floor of the primitive pharynx. In the adult this origin is marked by the foramen caecum. The caudal part of the hypobranchial region contributes with its epiglottal and the arytenoid swellings to the formation of the larynx.

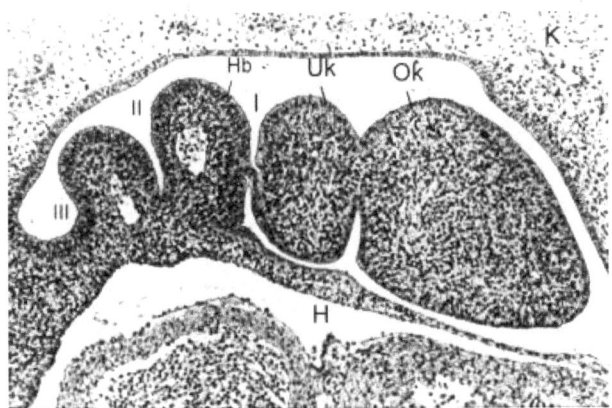

Fig.43: Cattle embryo, longitudinal section, xxHE: head mesenchyme (K), maxillary process (Ok), mandibular process (Uk), hyoid arch (Hb), I-III pharyngeal pouches, pericardial cavity (H).

Arch derivatives
The arch arteries connect dorsal and ventral aorta. The first, second and fifths are early reduced; the third, fourth and sixth are transformed to the carotids, aortic arch, subclavian, and pulmonary arteries (see cardivascular system). The nerves of arch 1-4 are listed above; the nerve of the fifth arch is the accessory nerve. The muscle blastema of the first arch is mainly for the masticatory muscles, of the second for facial muscles, of the following for pharyngeal and laryngeal muscles. The skeletal framework of the first and second arch are Meckel's cartilage (I), Reichert's cartilage (II) forming later malleus, incus and stapes. Material from arch 2-4 contributes to the larynx. The first cleft later forms the external acoustic meatus and the auricular hillocks. The closing membrane is the later tympanic membrane.

Pharyngeal pouch derivatives
The first pouch between first and second arch forms the tympanic cavity and the second pouch the tonsilar sinus. The third and fourth pouches are forming dorsally parathyroid blastems, ventrally thymus blastems. The fifth is reduced to a small recess for the ultimobranchial body, which stay separate in birds, but fuse with the thyroid gland in mammals forming its C-cells. In pig it is believed, that also the ectodermal cervical sinus contributes to the thymus. Differential growth and a different neck development produce species differences in the regional anatomy of these organs.

Head, neck and face development
The formation of head, neck und face is caused by the development of the

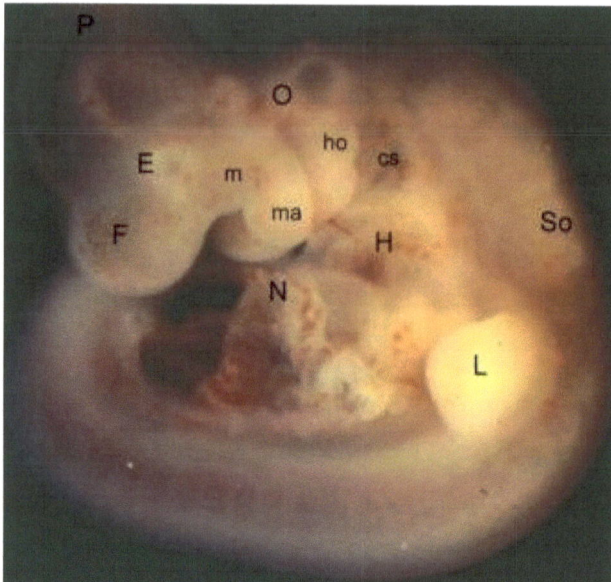

Fig.44: Cat embryo, 19 days, x: frontonasal process (F), parietal process (P), lens placode (E), otic vesicle (O), limb bud (L), somites (So), maxillary process (m), first cleft between the mandibular process (ma) of the first pharyngeal arch and the hyoid arch (ho), cervical sinus (cs).

brain vesicles, placodes and the transformation of the pharyngeal arches. Optic and otic placodes are already invaginated, the olfactory placode is transformed to a pit bounded by a medial and a lateral nasal process of the frontonasal prominence, the head is markedly flexed on the trunk at the parietal and cervical flexure, the hindbrain has a pontine flexure and a thin roof plate, the pharyngeal arches are more distict. Between the maxillary process, optic cup and the lateral nasal process the nasolacrimal duct is covered by ectoderm on both sides. The medial nasal process and maxillary processes are fusing to form the upper lip and maxilla, the mandibular processes fuse to form the lower lip and the mandibular. Different kind of cleft lips, palate and jaw are failures in fusion of these processes.

The caudal part of the hyoid arch is overlapping with the operculum the succeeding arches to enclose the cervical sinus; the cranial part with auricular hillocks around the external auditory meatus (from the first cleft) is forming the external ear. The mesenchyme of the arches and the hypobranchial region proliferate to develop the neck. There are important species differences, especially between birds and mammals. In birds the second arch mainly contributes to the neck, in mammals mainly the third arch, what causes differences in the regional anatomy of the adults. Now the typical species differences are distict.

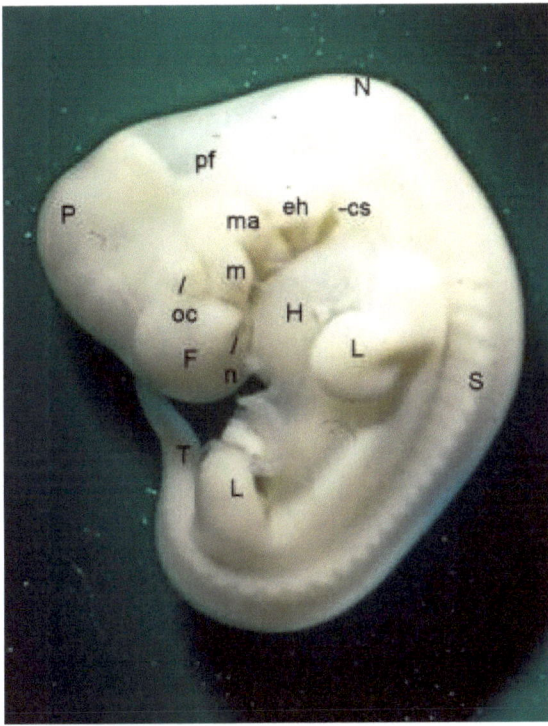

Fig.45: Cat embryo, 20 days, x: frontonasal - (F) and parietal prominence (P, cervical flexure (N), pontine flexure (pf), limb buds (L), tail (T), pericardial swelling (H), somites (S), nasal pit (n) with lateral and medial nasal processes, nasolacrimal duct between optic cup (oc), lateral nasal process and maxillary process (m), first cleft between mandibular process (ma) and auricular hillocks (eh), cervical sinus (cs).

Fig.46: Cat embryo, 22 days, x: the embryo with head, neck, limbs and tail is now species specific.

Oral cavity and teeth

Inside the oral cavity the tongue, the palate (see respiratory system), the salivary glands and teeth develop. The dental laminae develop as down growth of the surface ectoderm along the length of upper and lower jaw. From these ridges dental buds are separated on the labial surface for the temporary and on the lingual surface for the permanent teeth. These buds form caps (bell like) with an outer and

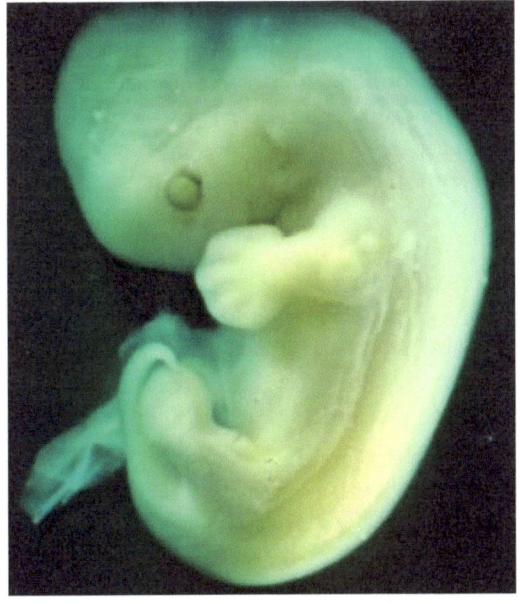

inner enamel epithelium and a core of stellate reticulum (ectodermal). The caps surround the dental (mesenchymal) papilla. The inner layer of the enamel epithelium differentiates to ameloblasts the mesenchyme next to it differentiates to odontoblasts. The surrounding mesenchyme is forming the root blastema with nerves and vessels and the maxillary and mandibular bone form alveolae around these tooth germs.

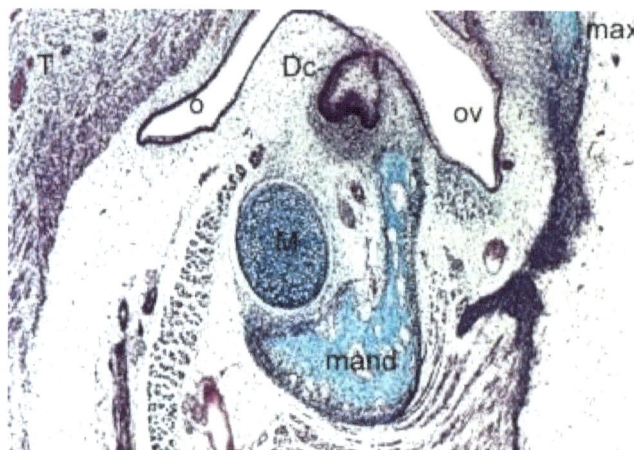

Fig.47: Tooth germ, cat embryo, 36 days, xxtrichrome: oral cavity (o), vestibulum (ov), maxillary bone (max), mandibular bone (mand), Meckel's cartilage (M), dental cap (Dc), tongue (T).

During fetal histogenesis the odontoblasts retreat into the dental papilla, leaving a thin dental process and produce throughout life predentine. The ameloblasts produce during fetal life enamel prisms and a dental cuticle from outside. The epithelial root sheath form the dentine for the growing teeth at the junction of the inner and outer enamel layer. Cementum is modified bone around the entire tooth in hypsodont teeth and at the root in brachydont teeth. Between the cementum und the alveolar bone develops the peridontal membrane from mesenchyme. There are many species differences.

Salivary glands

Beside small salivary glands, bigger glands like the parotid and the mandibular gland are initiated by epithelial invagination from the ectoderm of the oral cavity. This will later become the duct of these glands. Both duct branch dichotome up to day 36 (branching phase) into the surrounding mesenchyme. In the subsequent separation phase, smaller ducts and acini differentiate in primitive lobules, separated by early connective tissue. During fetal histogenesis intercalated and striated ducts are formed and mucous and serous cells start to produce complex carbohydrates in the acini.

Comparative Embryology

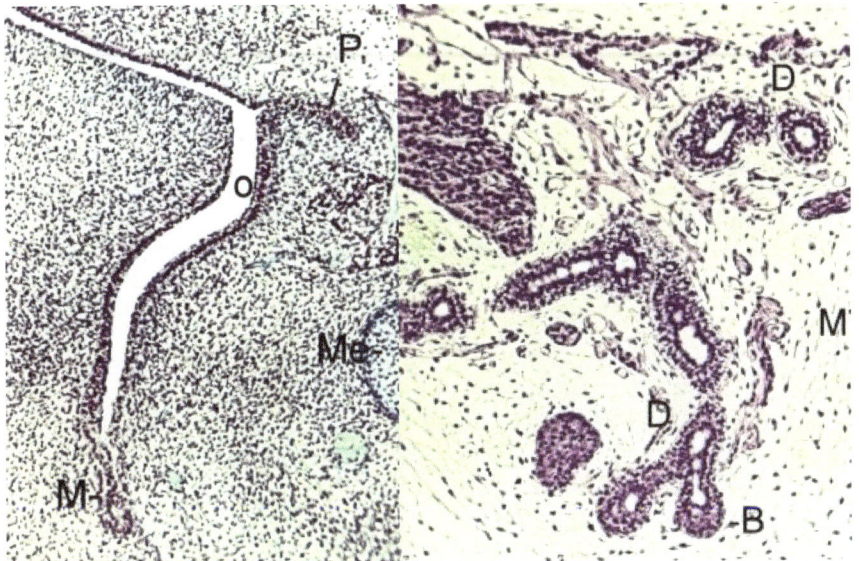

Fig. 48a (left side): oral cavity, cat embryo, 24 days, xxtrichrome: oral cavity (O), parotid duct (P), mandibular duct (M) as epithelial sprout, Meckel's cartilage (Me); **48b (right side):** mandibular gland, cat embryo, day 34, xxHE: ducts (D), acini (B), connective tissue (M).

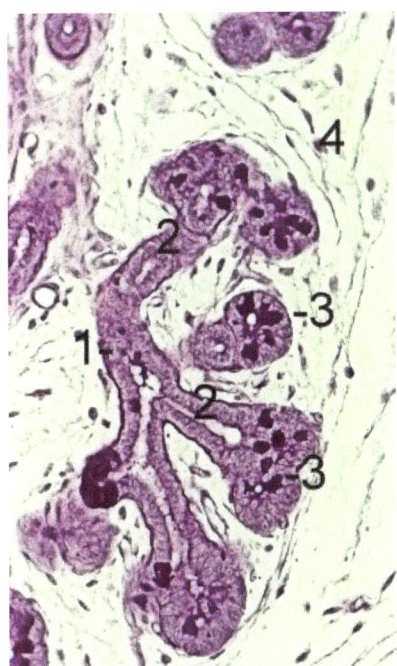

Fig.49: Mandibular gland, cat, fetus, prenatal, xxPAS: glandular ducts (1) glandular sprouts (2), and glandular acini mit PAS-postive cells surrounded by specific mesenchyme.

Esophagus and stomach

With the growth of the neck the foregut behind the primitive pharynx is rapidly elongating. The entoderm is the epithelial layer of this tubular esophagus; the surrounding mesenchyme forms all other layers. At its end a spindle shaped primitive stomach is formed with a dorsal great and a ventral lesser curvature attached by the dorsal and ventral mesogastrium to the body wall and the liver.

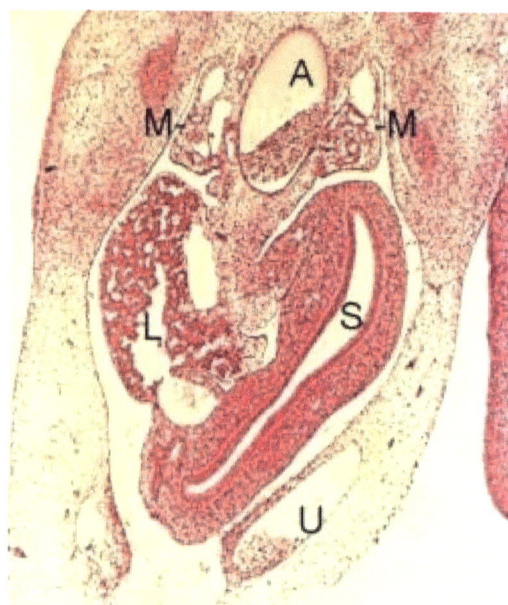

Fig. 50: Cat embryo, day 22, horizontal, xxHE: aorta (A), mesonephros (M), liver (L), stomach (S), umbilical vein (U).

By differential growth of the liver the greater curvature is turning caudally, the lesser curvature cranially, the inlet to the left and the outlet to the right. The dorsal mesogastrium is forced to elongate, forming a fold, the greater omentum with an extension of the peritoneal cavity called the omental bursa. In the dorsal mesogastrium the spleen develops. Its connection to the stomach transforms to the gastrolienal ligament. The ventral mesogastrium runs from the lesser curvature to the liver forming the floor of the vestibulum bursae, the entrance to which is at the level of its free border and is termed the epiploic foramen.

The various tunics of the stomach wall differentiate with day 19-24. First the gastric pits and glands are formed by the lining epithelium from day 24 on, about midterm, the primitive oxyntic and primitive mucous cells are formed. The latter is the precursor for all other cells, which differentiate during the fetal histogenesis. The secretion of the gastric proper glands starts shortly after birth. In many species the gastric surface epithelium produces a gastric lipase for a short period after birth. Pyloric stenosis sometimes occurs in kittens.

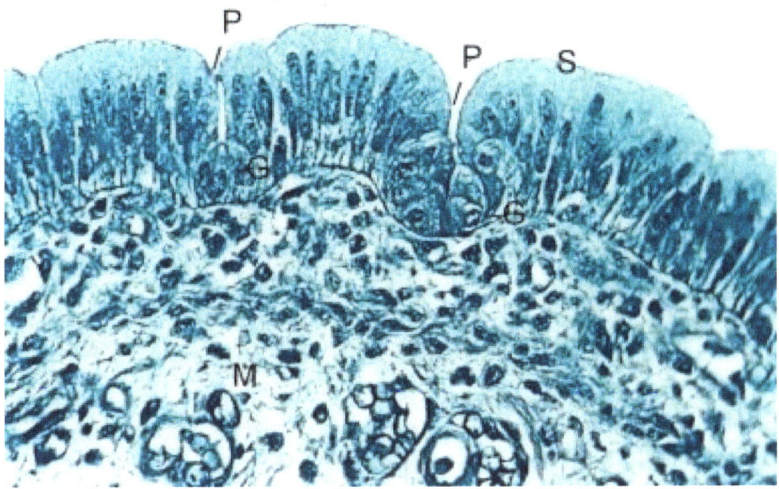

Fig. 51: stomach, cat embryo, day 24, xxxRichardson stain: stomach surface epithelium, primitive gastric pits (P), gastric glands (G), gastric mesenchyme(M).

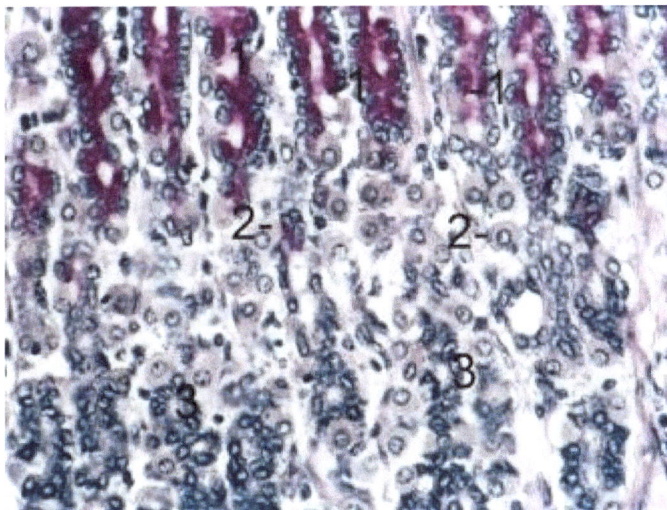

Fig.52: Proper glands of the stomach, prenatal cat fetus, xx Aurantia-PAS: mucous neck cells (1), oxyntic cells (2), peptic cells (3) in differentiation.

In ruminants the omentum is modified by the growth of the rumen, starting as a paired vesicle from the greater curvature. The omasum develops from the lesser curvature and the reticulum between rumen and omasum. The different compartments are oriented dorsoventrally, until a rotation of the rumen to the left occur. The greater omentum is attached with its lamellae

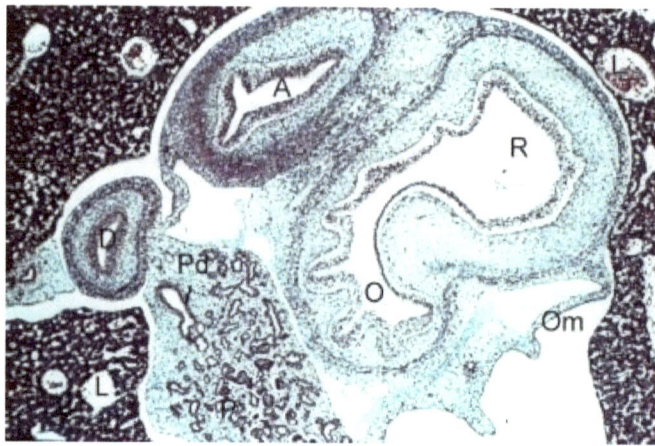

Fig.53: Stomach, sheep embryo, 3 cm CRL, xxtrichrome: abomasum (A), rumen (R), omasum (O), omentum (Om), duode-num (D), liver (L), pancreas (P), pancreatic duct (Pd).

to the longitudinal grooves of the rumen. Secondary changes in the arrangement of different organs in ruminants are due to the enlargement of the rumen. This includes attachment to the body wall, to the spleen and the shift of the left kidney to the right. The histogenesis of the specific surface projections like villi, cells and lamellae and all other layers are formed during the fetal periods.

Intestines

The rapid elongation of the midgut loop results in the physiological herniation into the umbilicus. Due to this elongation and the stomach

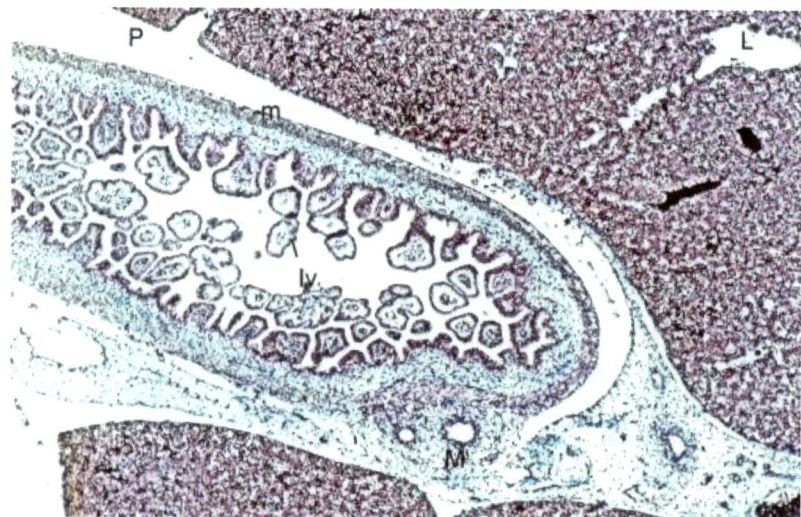

Fig. 54: Duodenum, cat embryo, day 34, xxtrichrome: peritoneal cavity (P), liver with blood islets (L), intestinal villi (Iv), muscle layer (m), mesenterium with blood vessels (M).

rotation the loop undergoes a right rotation around the cranial mesenteric artery (280-360°) forming a duodenal and a colonic hook. The differentiation of the ascending colon and caecal specialisation in pigs, ruminants and horses causes species differences. The histogenesis of all layer starts in the embryonal periods with the formation of villi, muscle layer and the serous membrane and continues during the fetal periods. Situs inversus is connected with a counter rotation of the gut. Persistence of the omphaloenteric duct leads to a gut fistula, a poor reduction of the duct is the Meckel's diverticulum.

The hindgut is the cloaca, the common termination closed by the cloacal membrane. The growth of the urorectal septum divides the cloaca into the anorectal canal, closed by the anal membrane, and ventral the perineum the urogenital sinus closed by the urogenital membrane. The urogenital sinus is connected to the allantois via the urachus. The urogenital sinus is later subdivided into a vesical, pelvic and phallic part (see urogenital system). A failure of the anal membrane to rupture (pig) is the anal atresia.

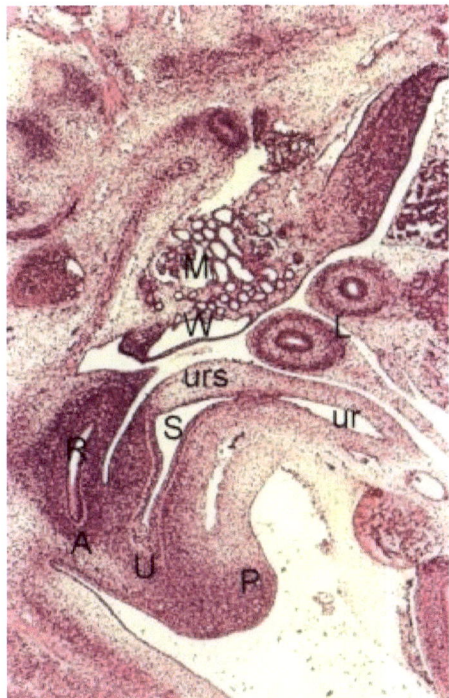

Fig. 55: Caudal part of a cat embryo, day 24, longitudinal section, xxHE: anal membrane (A), rectum (R), urogenital sinus (S), urogenital septum (U), phallus (P), urorectal septum (urs), urachus (ur), mesonephros (M), mesonephric duct (W), midgut loop (L).

Liver and Pancreas

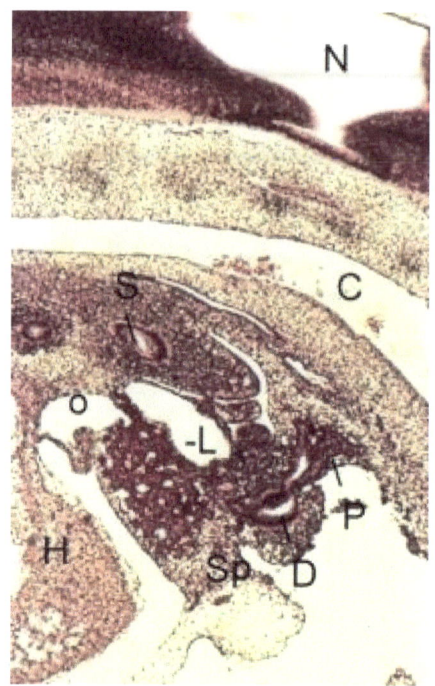

Behind the stomach the gut epithelium is growing into the septum transversum (also described as ventral mesogastrium), forming a shallow groove (plate) as rudiment of liver and biliary bladder. Epithelial sprouts of the liver rudiment invade the region of the omphalomesenteric vein and divide in this way caudal (Vv.hepaticae advehentes) and cranial hepatic (Vv. hepaticae revehentes) veins. Further branching creates hepatic cells cords surrounded by branches of the omphlomesenteric vein. During fetal histogenesis these structures are transformed to liver lobules and sinusoids.

Fig. 56: Cat embryo, day 19, longitudinal section, xxHE: neural tube (N), cardinal vein (C), heart (H), stomach (S), liver (L), dorsal pancreas diverticles (P), omphalomesenteric vein (O), septum transversum (Sp), duodenum (D).

The right umbilical and the left omphalomesenteric veins are later reduced. At the same time dorsal and ventral pancreatic diverticles from the midgut invaginate into the mesenteries forming ducts, acini and from the tip of the sprouts the endocrine islets. With the rotation of the intestines dorsal and ventral rudiments fuse.

The Respiratory Apparatus

The upper respiratory system develops together with the head and the pharynx. The olfactory (nasal) pit on both sides becomes deeper, forming a nasal sac, which is separated by the primary palate and more caudally by the bucconasal membrane from the oral cavity. In cat embryos of 19 days the bucconasal membranes rupture. From the maxillary processes two palatal processes and from the roof a nasal septum is growing downwards. With the tongue development these are united from rostrally to the secondary palate. Between primary palate and palatal processes the incisive fossa, and behind the choana is formed. With the fetal histogenesis, soft and hard palate with cartilage, bone and glands are developed. Anomalous fusion or lack of fusion results in cleft palate frequently associated with hare-lip. The paranasal sinuses develop postnatally from diverticles of the lateral nasal wall. At the end of the primitive pharynx directly behind the hypobranchial eminence the laryngotracheal groove is the rudiment of larynx, trachea and lungs. When the esophagus is growing the tracheaesophageal septum is separating the communication with the foregut, if not a tracheoesophageal fistula develops. Now the reduced communication is the primitive laryngeal aditus.

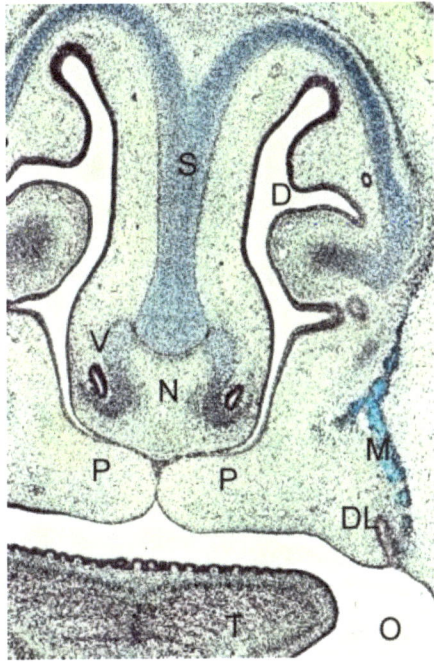

Fig.57: Cat embryo, 29 days, cross section of the head, xxtrichrome: palatal process (P) and nasal septum (N) are fusing, dental lamina (Dl), nasal diverticles (D), oral cavity (O), tongue (T), maxillary bone (M), vomeronasal organ (V).

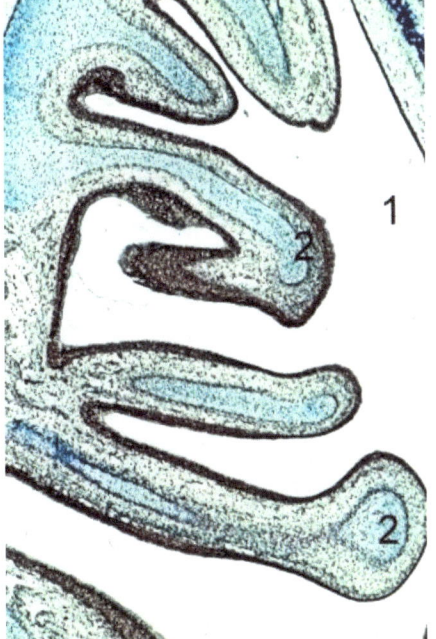

Fig.58: Nasal cavity, cat fetus 36 days, xtrichrom common nasal duct (1), chonchae (2).

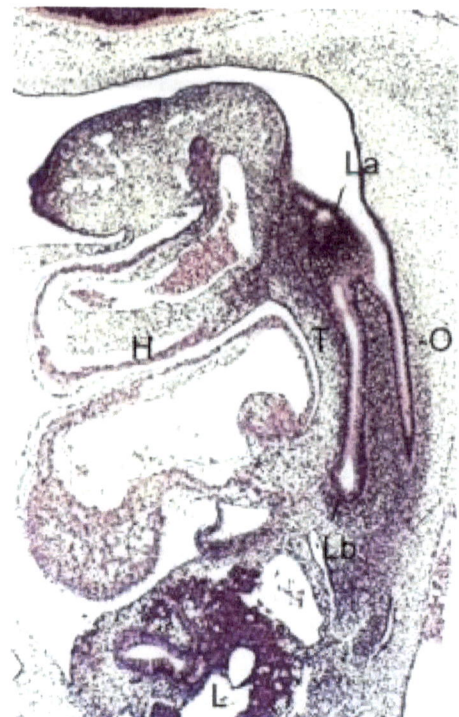

Fig.59: Cat embryo, 19 days, longitudinal section, xxHE: heart (H), liver (L), larynx (LA), lung bud (Lb), esophagus (O), trachea (T).

The caudal end of the pouch divides to the lung buds. Later this is the bifurcation of the trachea with the primary bronchi. The rostal part is forming the laryngeal cavity. The hypobranchial eminence will become the epiglottis. The lateral arytenoid swellings form the aryepiglottic folds and together with the pharyngeal derivatives the other cartilages of the larynx together with muscles. The tube elongates and differentiates to the trachea. The lung buds branch during the pseudoglandular stage into the bronchial tree and develop together with surrounding splanchnopleuric mesenchyme the lung inside the growing pleural cavity.

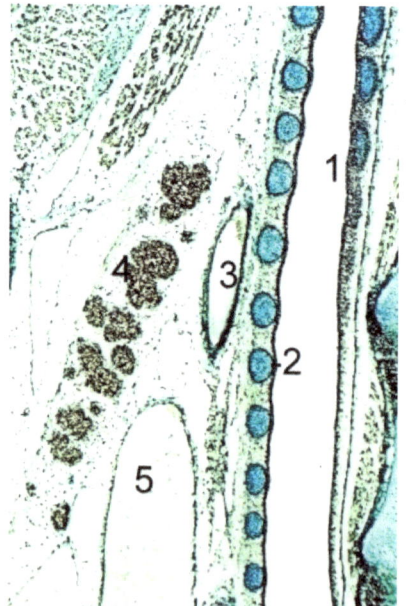

Fig.60: Trachea, cat fetus 36 days xx trichrome: lumen (1), cartilage of the trachea (2), A. carotis comm. (3) thymus (4), jugular vein (5).

Comparative Embryology

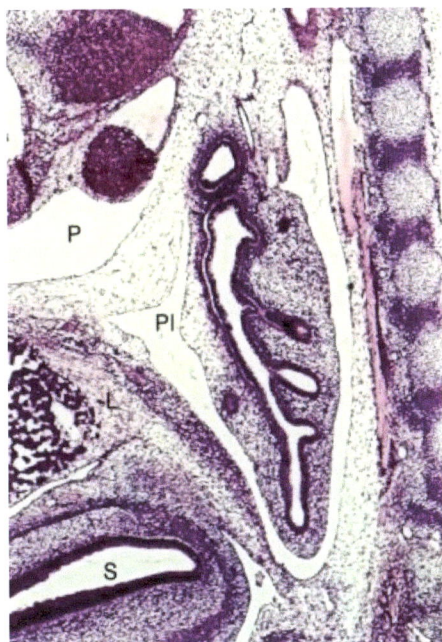

Fig.61: Cat embryo, 25 days, longitudinal section, xxHE: pseudo glandular lung in the pleural cavity (Pl), pericardial cavity (P), stomach (S).

Fig.62: Lungs, cat fetus 36 days, xx trichrome: bronchial (1), sprouts (2) in the late pseudoglandular stage.

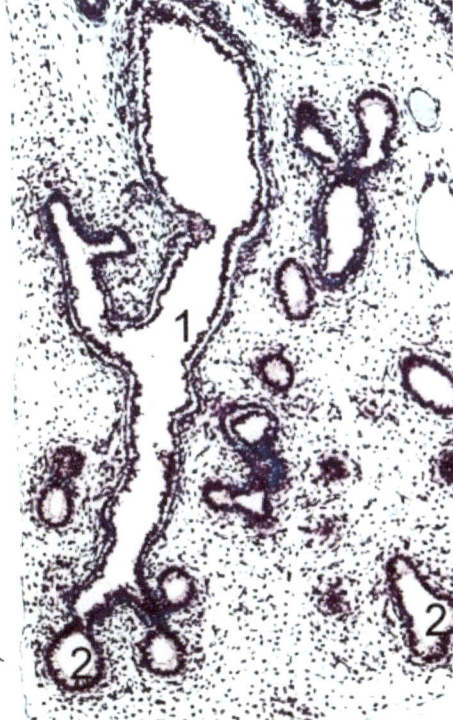

In the canalicular stage smaller bronchioli and in the terminal sac stage before birth the alveolar ducts are formed. The development of alveoli during the aveolar stage continues after birth. The surfactant production shortly before birth is a sign of the lung-maturation. This fails in the respiratory distress syndrome of newborns. The growing lobes of the lung enlarge also the pleural cavities, which are still in connection with the peritoneal cavity. During the early morphogenesis the mesentery of the esophagus develops from the pleuropericardial septum, which separates also the pleural and pericardial cavities. The mediastinum is formed by ventral growth of the pleural cavities and the connection of the two pleural sacs. The expanding peritoneal cavity is also forming the pneumato-enteric recesses on both sides of the esophagus. The left one soon disappears, the right one is the mediastinal cavity (Sussdorf) when separated from the peritoneal cavity or the infracardial bursa when open to the peritoneal cavity.

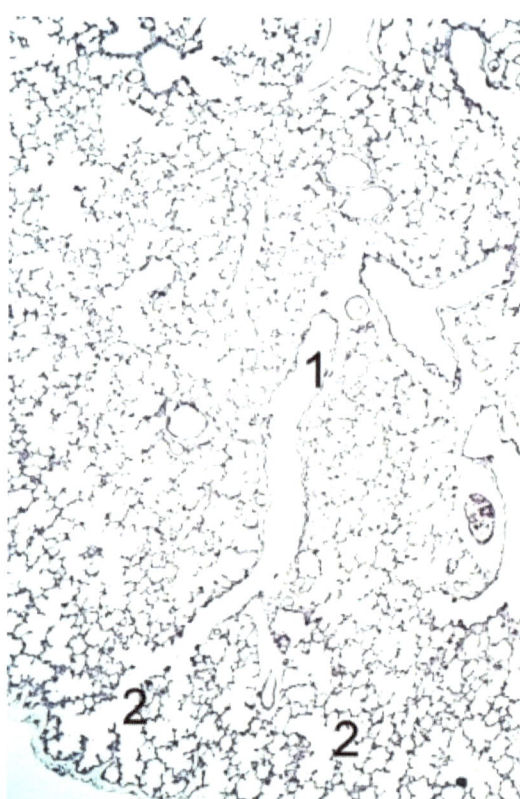

Fig.63: Lung, cat fetus 60 days x trichrome bronchial (1) und primitive alveolar ducts (2) in the alveolar stage.

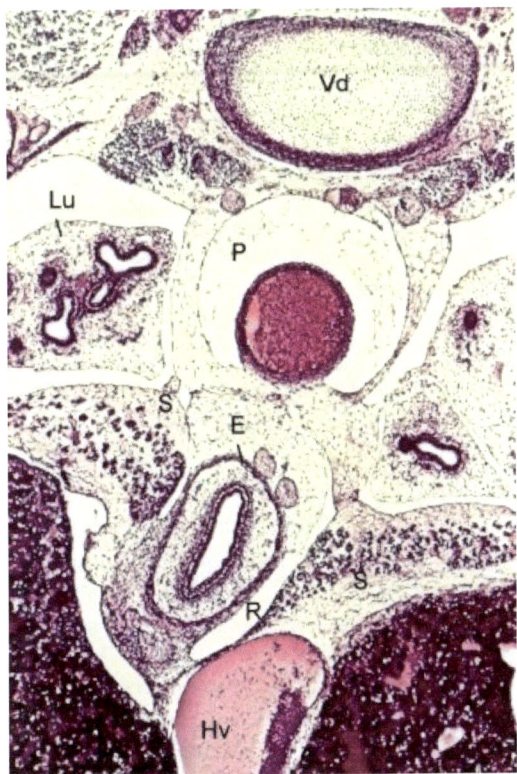

Fig. 64: Cat embryo, 31 days, cross section, xxtrichrome: esophagus (E) with the vagal nerve and a small left recess, left lung (Lu) in the pleural cavity, pericardio-peritoneal canal with the sinus venosus (P), septum transversum (S) with muscle blastem, hepatic vein (Hv) between the liver lobes, the right pneumatoenteric recess (R), blastem of the vertebral column.

The Urogenital Apparatus

The urinary system and the genital system are close related, originating from the intermediate mesoderm, which by the transverse folding of the embryo shifts ventrolaterally to the paraxial forming the unsegmented urogenital plate with a lateral nephrogenic ridge and a medial genital ridge. Both are covered by thicked coelomic epithelium. The somite stalk remains segmented and form nephrotomes. The unsegmented ridge forms the nephric duct. These differentiate to an excretion system of three different generations, the holonephros.

Kidney

The first generation is a rudimentary organ, pronephros, in mammals, only visible in early somite stages and most cranial situated in segment 4-14, with one nephrostoma and a simple canal per segment induced by the ridge. These segments have an outer glomerulum supplied by the dorsal aorta. The pronephric duct is ending in the hindgut transforming it to the cloaca. The pronephros is only in primitive vertebrates like cyclostomata a functional kindney, but transitory in mammals.

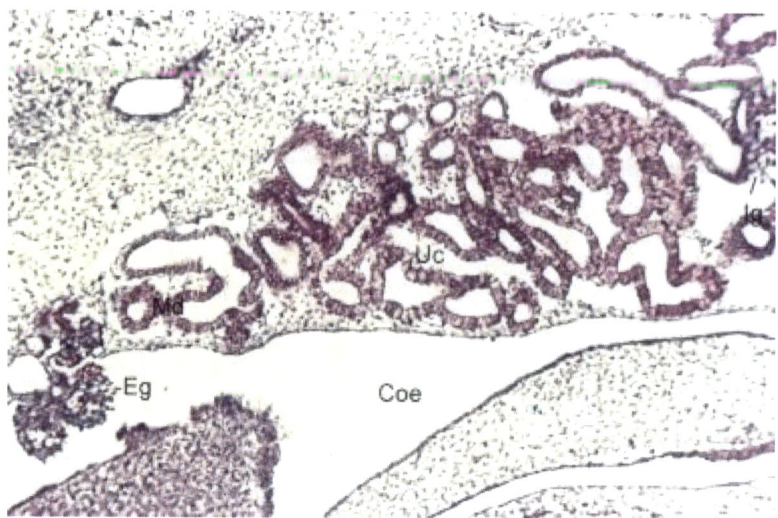

Fig.65: Cat embryo, 19 days, longitudinal section, xxtrichrome: external glomerula (Eg) of the pronephros, internal glomerula (Ig) of the mesonephros, mesonephric tubules (Uc), mesonephric duct (Md), coeloma (Coe).

The mesonephros develops caudal to the pronephros, from segment 14-30, with 1-3 S-shaped tubules per segment with a secretory and a collective part induced by the mesonephric duct. This kidney has inner glomerula with capsules. The former pronephric duct is used as the mesonephric duct (Wolffian duct). It is the kidney for amphibians and fish, but a huge transitory organ in mammals forming the inner mesonephric fold and the outside mesonephric ridge. It is active in sheep and pig embryos during the first trimester. In the early fetus it undergoes involution. In all mammals remnants of the organ are important for the development of the genital organs.

The metanephros develops from the unsegmented metanephric blastem dorsal between segment 29-31 and the ureteric bud, a dorsal invagination of the distal part of the mesonephric duct. It is the permanent kidney in all amniots. The bud is dividing dichotome, growing into the metanephric blastem and inducing several generations of nephrogenic corpuscles, which form all elements of the nephrons like glomerula and tubules. In this way all collecting are derivatives from the ureteric bud, all tubules and glomerula are derivatives from the metanephric blastem. During the fetal histogenesis all elements differentiate. Later the tubules and the collecting ducts fuse. There are many species differences in the number of generations, in the way of nephron formation, size of corpuscles, length and orientation of the tubules, size of renal pyramids, calyx formation from collecting ducts and

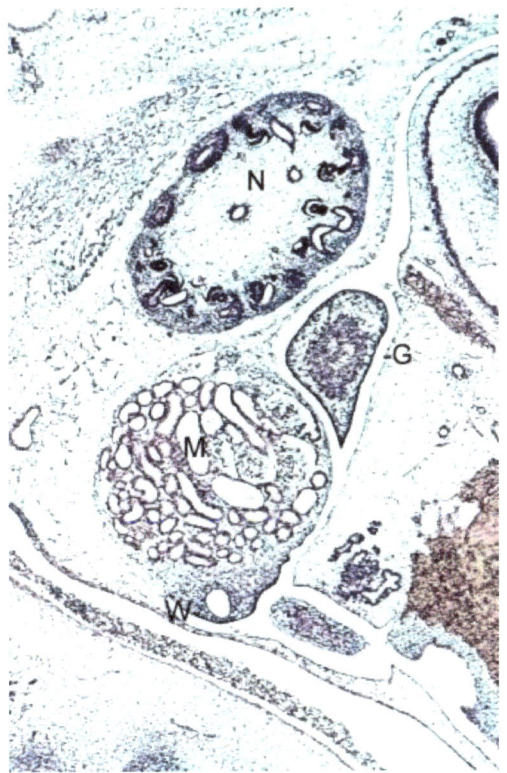

Fig.66: Cat embryo, 25 days, longitudinal section, xx trichrome: metanephros (N) with the first generation of nephrogenic corpuscles, the degenerating mesonephros (M), mesonephric duct (W), gonad (G).

the surface fusion of the fetal primary lobes. Already embryonal the specific circulatory system is developed. By the reduction of the mesonephros, the metanephric growth and the development of the caudal body part the kidneys ascend up to the adrenal bodies. Ruminal development in ruminants causes a secondary shift of the left kidney to a middle intraabdominal position. Malformations are renal agenesis, non ascent of kidneys and congenital cystic kidney, when nephrons and collecting tubules not connected.

Fig.67: Cat embryo, 33 days, cross section of the metanephros, xx HE: collecting ducts (cd) divide dichotome and induce nephrogenic corpucles of the first (fc), second (sc) and third (tc) generation, metanephric blastem (mB), from these primitive glomerula (gl) and nephric tubules (t) develop.

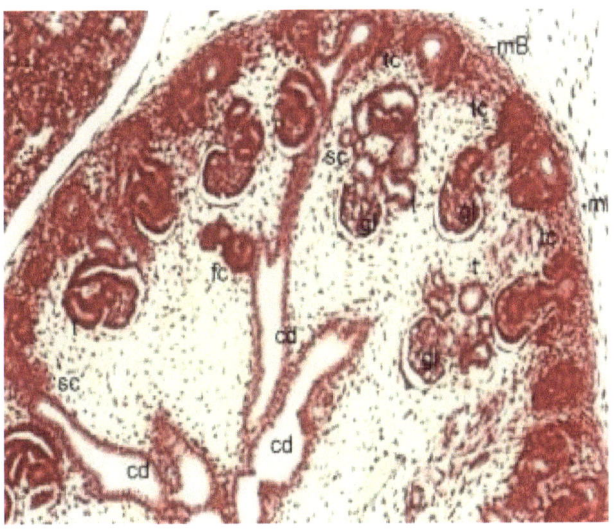

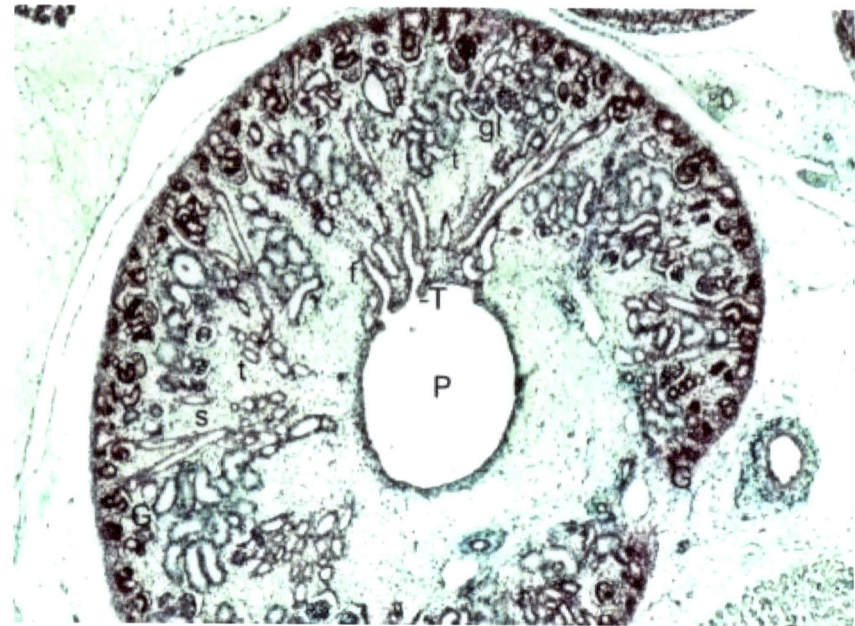

Fig.68: Cat embryo, 36 days, cross section of the metanephros, xxtrichrome: primitive pelvis (P), collecting duct (T), dichotome division of the ducts of the first (f) and second generation (s), inducing nephrogenic corpuscles (G), which are developing glomerula (gl) and tubuli (t).

Ureter, Urinary bladder and Urethra

The ureter is formed from the distal part of the ureteric bud ending via the mesonephric duct into the urogenital sinus, when the urorectal septum has divided the cloaca. The terminal part of the mesonephric duct forms a vesical trigone in the expanding sinus wall. By differential growth the ureter later opens directly into the vesical part of the sinus, which will form most of the urinary bladder during fetal histogenesis (the trigone is mesonephric material). The pelvic part of the sinus forms the female urethra and the pelvic part of the male urethra. The phallic part of the sinus forms the penile part of the urethra in the male. The cranial part of the sinus is still connected with the allantois via the urachus. After birth the urachus is reduced inside the median ligament of the bladder.

Fig.69(next page): Cat embryo, 29 days, cross section, xxtrichrome: mesonephros (M), rectum (R), mesonephric duct (W), paramesonephric duct (M), ureter (U), urogenital sinus (S), umbilical artery (uA).

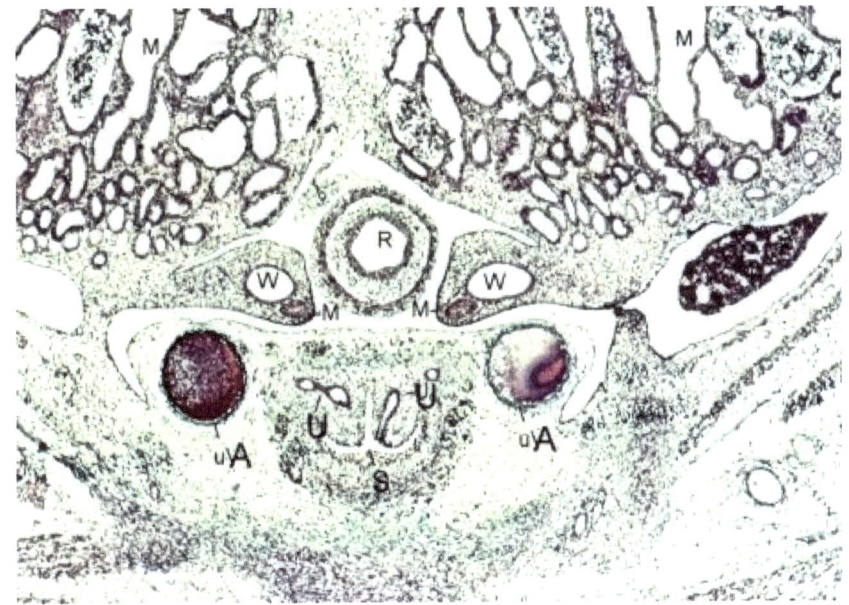

The Genital Apparatus

The gonads develop from the genital ridges medial of the mesonephros. At these sides the covering coelomic epithelium is thickened (germinativ epithelium) containing the primordial germ cells (PGC), which originate from the yolk sac. The mesenchyme underneath is forming a dense blastema, including material from the mesonephros. This is the indifferent stage of the gonads. The transformation of the gonads to a specific stage is induced by the primordial germ cells.

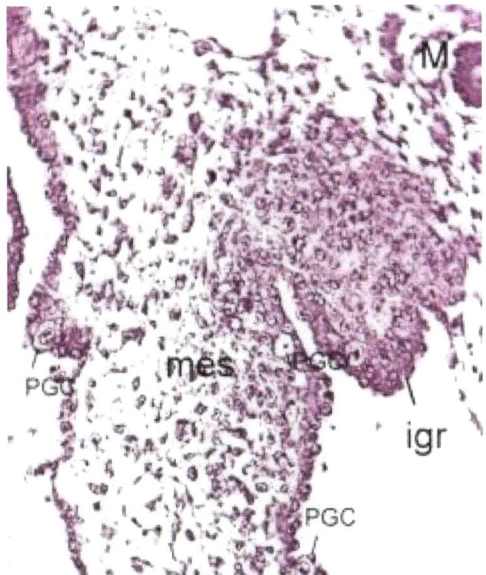

Fig.70: Cat embryo, 19 days, cross section, xxHE: indifferent genital ridge (igr), mesonephros (M), mesenterium (mes), primordial germ cells (PGC).

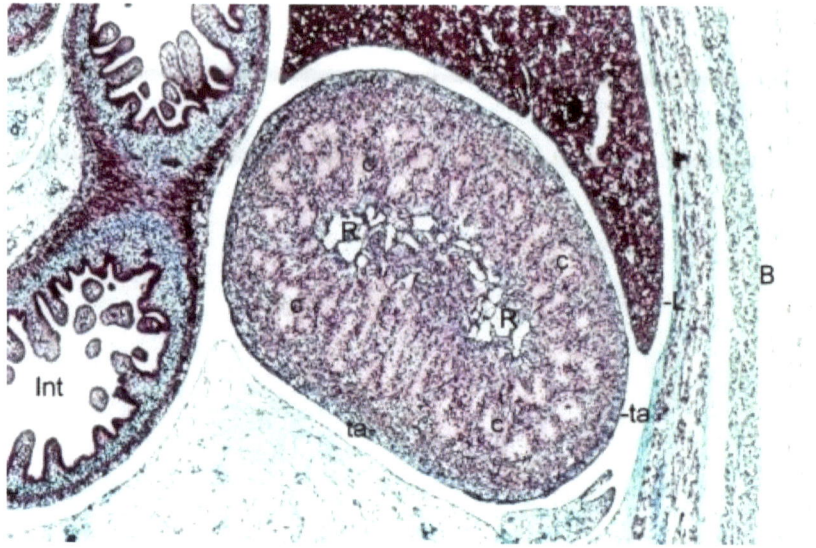

Fig. 71: Cat embryo, 36 days, cross section, xxtrichrome: intestines (Int), liver (L), body wall (B), medullary cords (c), rete (R), tunica albuginea (ta).

The Male Genital Apparatus

Under influence of the testicular determining factor (TDF) primitive sex cords proliferate deep into the gonad forming medullary cords, which are separated from the surface by the developing tunica albuginea. Mesonephric tubules form the rete and efferent ductuli, remnants of the mesonephros are also transformed to the epididymis. The cords with sertoli precoursors and primordial germ cells form the primitive seminiferous tubules. The primordial germ cells proliferate to produce spermatogonia, which rest until pubertal meiosis. Clusters of interstitial cells produce androgens to stimulate the further development of the male genital system. The peritoneal cover of the regressing mesonephros, the urogenital fold, is the mesentery of the gonads with different parts: the cranial diaphragmatic ligament, the middle mesorchium and the caudal inguinal ligament, which act as gubernaculum of the testis, because it connects testis and epididymis with the scrotal swellings. During the formation of the vaginal process this gubernaculum is shortened under the influence of androgens, producing the testical descent before birth in ruminants, around birth in horses and pigs and after birth in cat and dog.

The Male Duct System

Important for the duct system is the transformation of the mesonephros and the mesonephric duct. Medial from this duct the paramesonephric

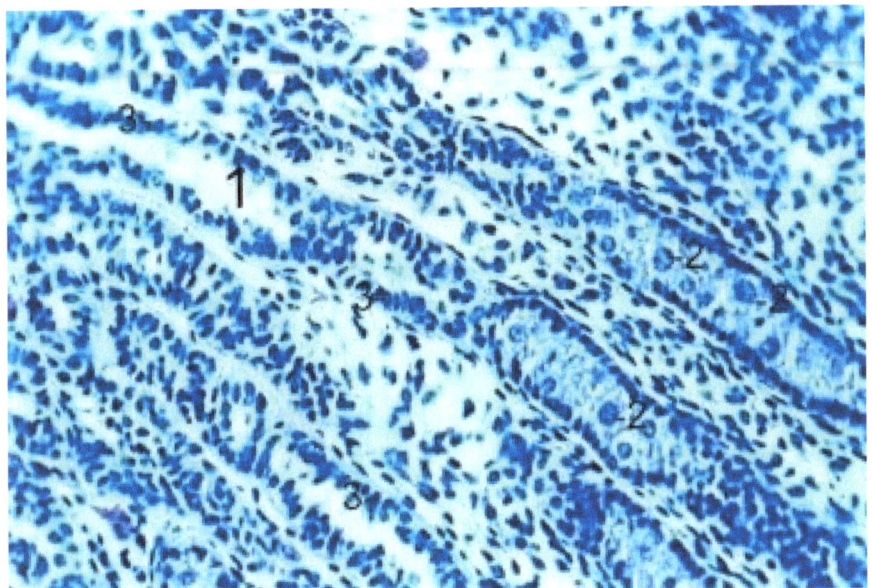

Fig.72: Testis, cat fetus, prenatal, xxRichardson: primitive tubuli (1) with spermatogonia (2) and supporting cells (3).

(Müllerian) duct is induced. These ducts appear in both sexes, one on each side, but attain complete development only in the female. In the male androgens stimulate the growth of the mesonephric ducts and the muellerian inhibiting factor cause the regression of the paramesonephric ducts. Remnants of the paranephric ducts in the male are the utriculus prostaticus or the male uterovagina. Former mesonephric tubules are transformed to the efferent ductules connecting the rete with the epididymal duct, which is formed by the former mesonephric duct. Sometimes additional mesonephric tubules persist as paragenital or paradidymal appendix. The distal part of the mesonephric duct is transformed to the deferent duct, which ends in the phallic part of the urogenital sinus. The distal part of the duct is also the material for the ampulla, the vesicular gland and the ejaculatory duct (mesodermal). The prostate gland is an outgrowth of the pelvic division of the sinus (endodermal), and the bulbourethral gland develops from the phallic part of the urogenital sinus (endodermal). The preputial diverticle of pigs is part of the ectodermal genital tubercle.

The Female Genital Apparatus

Also in the female gonad primitive cords are growing, but they disappear in the medulla or may form interstitial cells. Secondary, short cortical cords arise from the coelomic epithelium and form cell clusters of proliferating oogonia and epithelial cells. These oogonia enter the first meiotic division forming primary oocytes covered by follicular epithelial cells in several million primordial follicles. The oogenesis is arrested at the dictyotene stage of the prophase, which allows the oocyte a reduced metabolism. The cyclic folliculogenesis normally starts with puberty. In some species, including the cat there is an acyclic folliculogenesis possible, depening on the hormone stituation. But more than 99% of the primordial follicles are lost by atresia.

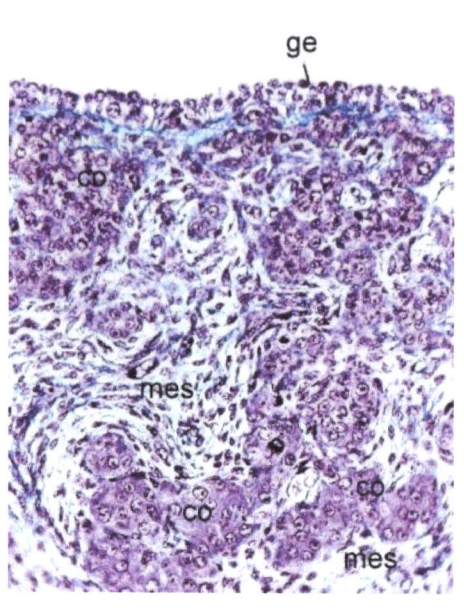

Fig. 73: Ovary, cat embryo, 33 days, xxtrichrome: germinal epithelium (ge), cortical cords (co), mesenchyme (mes).

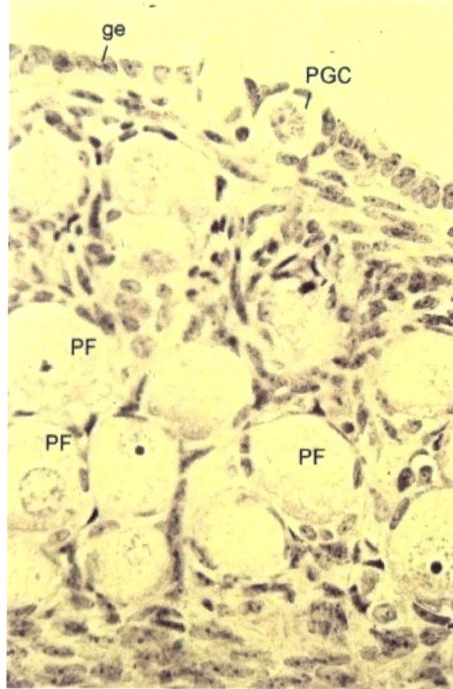

Fig.74: Ovary, cat, newborn, xxxHE: germinal epithelium (ge), primordial germ cell (PGC), primordial follicles (PF).

The Female Duct System

The female duct system develops mainly from the paranephric ducts, which invaginate from the coeloma, induced by the mesonephric ducts. Estrogens stimulate their growth and differentiation. The cranial parts later form the uterine tube, the middle parts the uterine horns and the caudal parts fuse and form the uterine body and neck and the proximal part of the vagina in a

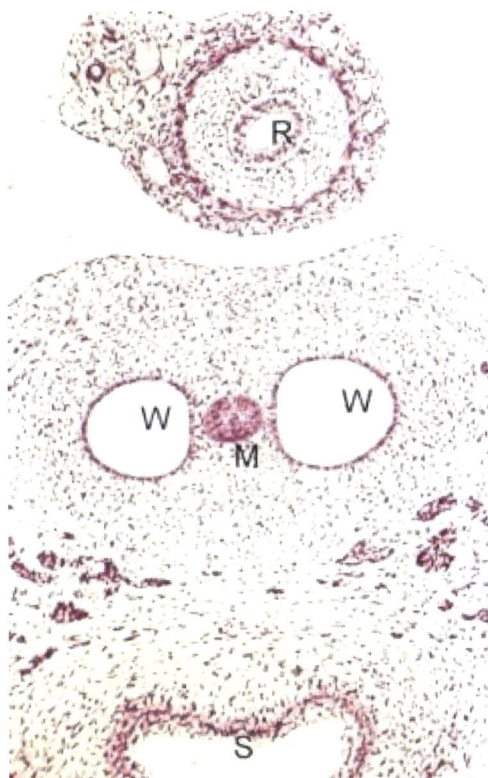

species specific pattern. The other part of the vagina is formed by the entodermal sinovaginal bud (or plate) from the pelvic part of the urogenital sinus. This plate is later visible as hymen and vaginal vestibule. The pelvic part and the phallic part of the sinus contribute in different ways (species depending) to the distal part of the vestibule.

Fig.75: Cat embryo, cross section of the caudal plica urogenitalis, xxHE: rectum (R), mesonephric duct (W), fused paramesonephric ducts (M), urogenital sinus (S).

The External Genitals

In the early, indifferent stage there are in both sexes around the cloacal membrane three small protuberances: the genital (phallic) tubercle in front and the genital (labioscrotal) swellings flanking the membrane.

Fig.76: Cat embryo, 25 days, longitudinal section, xxtrichrome: vertebral column (V), rectum (R), phallus (P), anal membrane (A), urogenital membrane (U), urethral groove (UR).

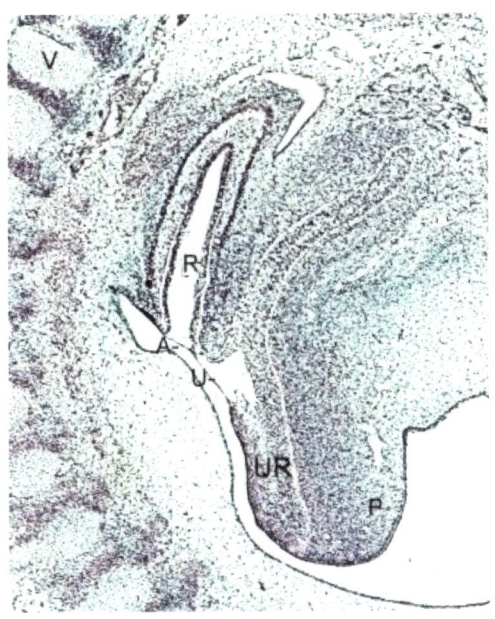

During the subdivision of the cloaca (see hindgut) the genital tubercle proliferates to the phallic tubercle (phallus), and the cloacal membrane is subdivided into the caudal anal membrane and the rostral urogenital membrane or urethral groove, which is flanked by the epithelial urethral folds. Soon the urogenital membrane opens forming the definitive urethral groove, the phallic part of the sinus. In the male fetus definitive folds are later closed in the midline forming the raphe leaving only the primitive urogenital orifice open. In the female fetus these stay open and the genital swellings remain separate and flank the base of the phallus, whereas in the male the genital swellings become rounded, migrate caudally and fuse to form the scrotum. The prepuce develops as an ingrowth of epithelium and inside the now established penis the cavernose bodies are formed. The failure of fusion of the the urethral folds is known as hypospadia. Due to hormonal factors many malformations occurs like hermaphrodits or freemartin, a heifer with depressed female organ development due to conjoined placentae. Cryptorchidism is a failure of the testicular descent (could be abdominal or inguinal, uni- or bilateral).

The Nervous System

Already after gastrulation the neural plate is induced by the notochord (see above). Now neural ectoderm is determined and differs from the rest of the ectoderm. With the neurulation process this plate is invaginated for the formation of the neural tube, the brain vesicles and the neural crests. The closure of the tube commences in the head region and leaves only a cranial and caudal opening. Cranial the tube is dilatated to the first brain vesicle, the archencephalon. Very soon a second vesicle, the deuteroencephalon is formed.

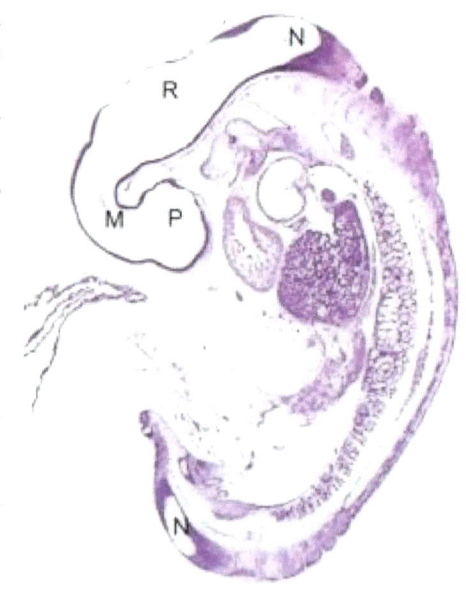

Fig.77: Pig embryo, 6 mm, longitudinal section, xHE: prosencephalon (P), mesencephalon (M) with midbrain flexure, rhombencephalon (R) with a thin roof, neural tube (N) with neck and rump flexure.

Due to elongation over the notochord the rostral vesicle turns ventrally. In the flexure a third vesicle occurs. This produce three expanded vesicles now termed forebrain- (prosencephalon), midbrain- (mesencephalon) and hindbrain- (rhombencephalon) vesicle with a midbrain flexure in between and a cervical flexure at the end. At this stage the lining neuroepithelium is already differentiated into neuroblasts and glioblasts. The forebrain vesicle is soon laterally outpouching and forming an unpaired diencephalic vesicle with dorsolateral telencephalic vesicles and ventrolateral optical vesicles on both sides. Behind the midbrain vesicle a pontine flexura divides the hindbrain into a metencephalic and a myelencephalic part.

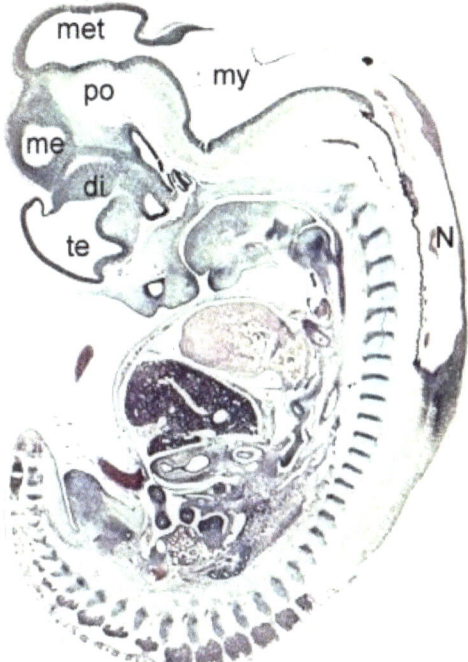

Fig.78: Sheep embryo, 28 days, longitudinal section, xHE: telencephalon (te), diencephalon (di), mesencephalon (me), metencephalon (met), myelencephalon (my), pontine flexure (po), neural tube (N).

The neuroblasts of the neural tube start to outgrow processes which lie mainly in the peripheral region. In this way a mantle zone with the nerve cell bodies and a marginal zone with their processes is formed. Uneven growth of the developing neural tube leads to formation of the relatively thick lateral plates and thin dorsal and ventral plates. The lumen of the tubes is the smaller central canal. A groove on the lateral wall of the cavity of the tube is termed the sulcus limitans and demarcates the dorsal zone as the alar lamina and the ventral zone as the basal lamina. By further dorsomedial and ventrolateral growth a dorsal median septum and ventral median fissure are formed. Outside the neural crests produce a line of spinal ganglia. Their neuroblasts later connect to the alar plate of the spinal cord. The growing marginal zone is later the white matter. The mantle zone is later the gray matter. In the white matter the ascending and descending pathways, in the gray matter the afferent and efferent cell columns are established and connected to peripheral structures.

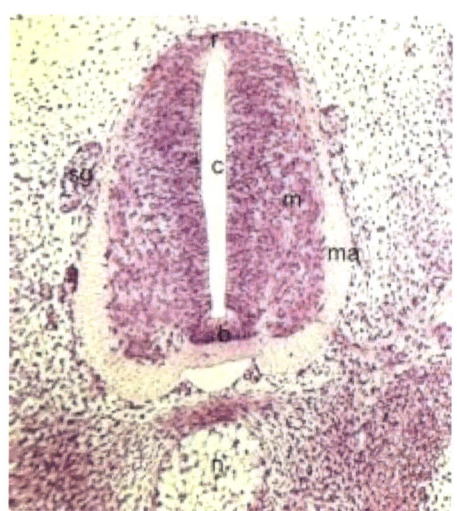

Fig.79: Neural tube, cat embryo, 21 days, cross section, xxHE: basal plate (b), roof plate (r), central canal (c), mantle zone (m), marginal zone (ma), notochord (n).

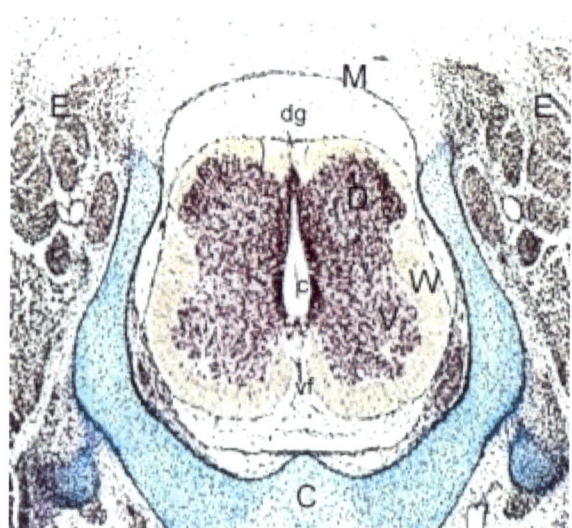

Fig.80: Spinal cord, cat embryo, 30 days, xxtrichrome: epaxial muscles (E), vertebrae (C), alar plate (D), basal plate (V), white substance with glial septum (dg), ventral fissure (vf), primitive meninges (M), marginal zone (W).

All parts of the peripheral nervous system are formed by the neural crest, which is also responcibile for the mesectoderm of the head, different ganglia, melanocytes, different endocrine cells, satellite cells, Schwann cells, the adrenal medulla and odontoblasts.

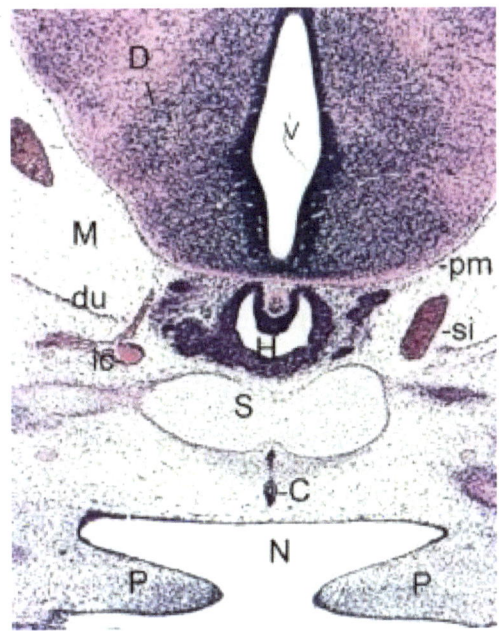

Fig.80: Diencephalon of the cat, 34 days, cross section, xxHE: diencephalic nuclei (D), third ventricle (V), primitive pia (pm), archnoid (M), dura (du), hypophysis (H), cranial sinus (si), internal carotid (ic), presphenoidal cartilage (S), craniopharyngeal duct (C), nasopharynx (N), secondary palate (P).

During the fetal histogenesis the different neurons and glia cells are differentiated. First the neural cord is approximately equal in length to the vertebral column. Due to differential growth the vertebral column exceeds that of the cord, what produces a virtual medullary ascend, forming the cauda equina and the termination of the cord between lumbal and sacral vertebrates depending on the species. From the surrounding mesenchyme the primitive meninges and from the somite sclerotomes vertebral cartilages are formed.

Also the brain is growing and differentiating glia and neurons. Inside the ventricles the choroid plexus is formed, already producing fluid. Overproduction or blockage of the resorption leads to hydrocephalus. First there are similar column in the caudal parts of the brain, but during the fetal histogenesis additional columns and nuclei are formed. The cortex of the forebrain is growing and differentiating, but still smooth, whereas the cortex of the cerebellum starts already with surface folding. For details of the complicated histogenesis see the specific literature. Like spinal nerves also the cranial nerves are made of neural crest material. Additionally for the ganglia of the cranial nerves there are different ectodermal placodes dorsally from the pharyngeal arches. Two cranial nerves are exceptional in the development of afferent neurons. The afferent neurons of the olfactory nerve develop from the nasal placode and connect secondarily with the olfactory bulb, and the optic nerve develops from the optic vesicle of the diencephalon. The material for the other cranial nerves is mesectodermal from periorbital, pharyngeal and hypobranchial origin.

Sense Organs

Eye and ear commence with ectodermal placodes, the lens placode and the ear placode. The lens placode is induced by the optic vesicle, a lateral outgrowth from both sides of the future diencephalic vesicle. The otic placode, which invaginate to the otic vesicle, is induced by the hindbrain vesicle.

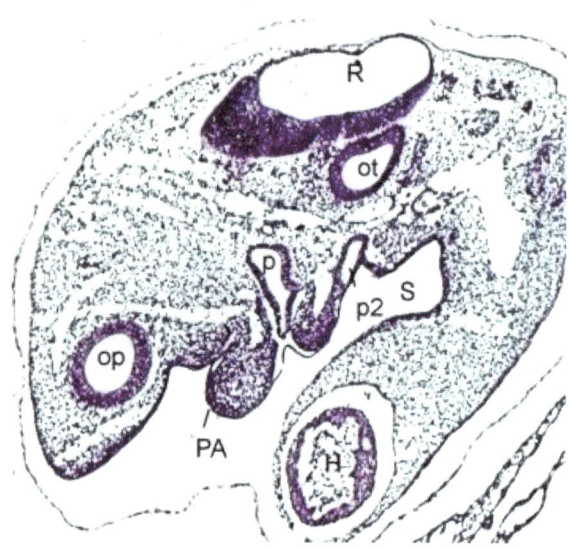

Fig.81: Cat embryo, 19 days, surface, longitudinal section, xHE: rhombencephalic vesicle (R), otic pit (ot), optical vesicle (op) from the forebrain, first pharyngeal arch (PA), first pharyngeal pouch, second pharyngeal pouch (p2), stomodaeum (S), heart (H).

The visual apparatus

The optic vesicle then becomes a proximal elongated part, the optic stalk and a distal dilated double-layered part, the optic cup, which is closely related to the invaginating lens placode. The depressed lens placode is then converted into a vesicle, separated from the surface ectoderm. The optic cup is incomplete at the choroidal fissure. Its wall gives origin to the retina, ciliary body and iris. The hyaloid artery passes along the choroidal fissure covered later with mesenchyme. Nonfusion of the fetal fissure results in a colo-boma. The outer layer of the cup becomes the pigmented layer of the retina and the inner layer of the cup is differentiating during the fetal period into the nervous layers of the retina. Between the inner layer and the lens is mesenychme forming the hyaloid substance. The distal part of the hyloid artery regresses, its proximal part is the central retinal artery. Surrounding mesenchyme is forming the choroid and the sclera. The outer ectoderm is forming the cornea and the eyelids. The aqueous chamber arises as a cavity in the mesenchyme in front of the lens.

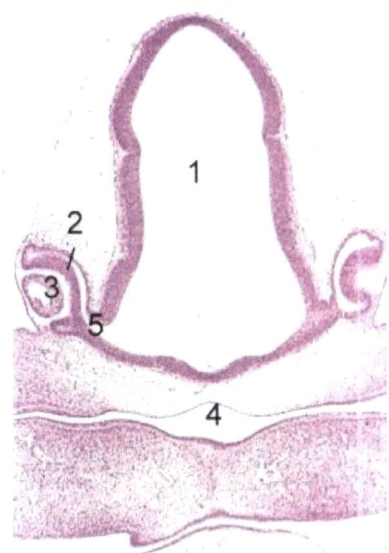

Fig.82: Sheep embryo, 15 mm CRL, cross section, xHE: diencephalon (1), optic cup (2), lens vesicle (3), primitive pharynx (4), optic stalk (5).

Later the chamber is separated by the ciliary body. The ectodermal epithelium of the lens vesicle produce elongated fibres which progressively fill the cavity of the vesicle forming the nucleus of the lens. The surface ectoderm is reconstituted to form the corneal epithelium. Accessory structures of the eye, conjunctiva, muscles, and the lacrimal glands develop during the fetal period. The eyelids develop as skin folds above and below the eye. When formed they then fuse together, thereby closing the palpebral fissure. In some species the margins of the lids separate again prior to birth but in pups and kittens this does not occur until several days after birth.

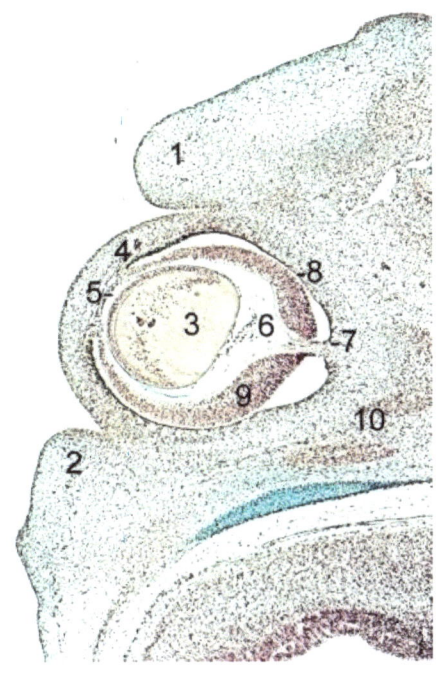

Fig.83: Cat embryo, 25 days, cross section, xtrichrome: upper- (1), lower lid (2), lens (3), cornea (4), aqueous chamber (5), vitreous body (6), optic stalk (7), outer layer of the optic cup (8), inner layer of the optic cup (9), blastem of eye muscles (10).

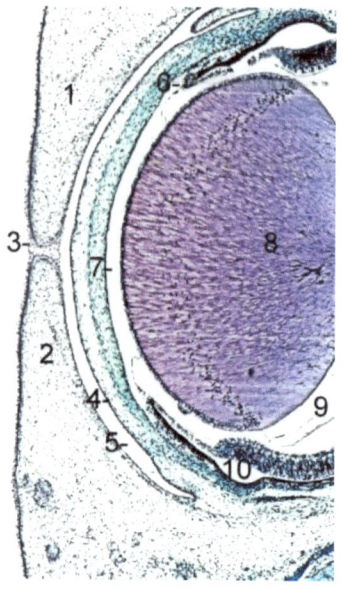

Fig.84: Cat embryo, 33 days, cross section, xtrichrome: upper- (1), lower lid (2), fused eyelid margins (3), cornea (4), conjunctival sac (5), iris (6), aqueous chamber (7), lens (8), vitreous humor (9), retina at the ciliary body (10).

The auditory apparatus

The external ear is formed the auricular hillocks in the dorsal region of first pharyngeal arch. The external acoustic meatus develops from the 1st pharyngeal cleft. The closing membrane develops the tympanic membrane with an outer ectodermal epithelium and inner endodermal epithelium. During the development the membrane is thickend with mesenchyme. The 1st pharyngeal pouch produces the auditory tube and the tympanic cavity. Malleus and incus are derivatives of the 1st and the stapes of the 2nd arch. The muscles of the middle ear are from the first and second arch material.

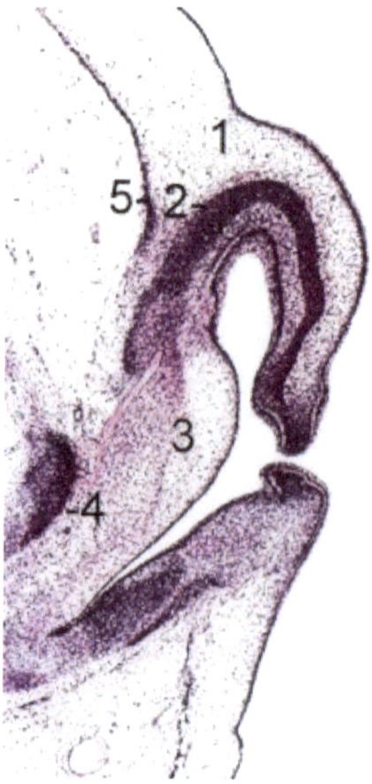

Fig.85: Cat embryo, 33 days, cross section, x HE: external ear (1), auricular cartilage (2), tympanic membrane (3), malleus blastem (4), tympanic ring (5).

Comparative Embryology

The internal ear is formed by the otic placode, which is invaginated to the otic pit. Later it becomes separated from the surface to form the otic vesicle or otocyst. Neural crest material establishes the primordium of the acoustic-facial ganglion, which is later separated into the facial and the vestibulo-cochlear ganglion. The otocyst is constricted into an upper vestibular pouch and a lower cochlear pouch and from the medial wall an endolymphatic sac is outpouched. From the vestibular pouch the semicircular ducts are formed, from the cochlear pouch the saccule and the rapidly elongating cochlea duct are formed. The histogenesis of these primitive elements starts during the fetal period.

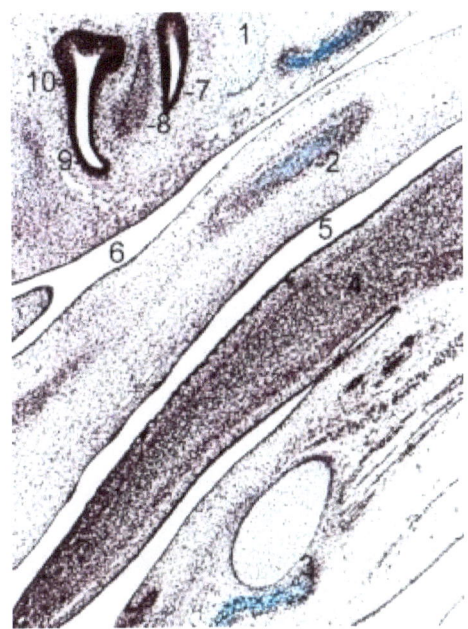

Fig.86: Cat embryo, 36 days, cross section, xtrichrome: blastem of the petrosum (1), palate with maxilla (2), Meckel's cartilage and mandible (3), tongue (4), oral cavity (5), nasopharynx (6), semicircular canal (7), vestibulocochlear ganglion (8), cochlear duct (9), saccule (10).

The olfactory apparatus

The olfactory (nasal) placodes become depressed to form the olfactory pits. At the fundic part of the nasal cavity the olfactory epithelium transform into neuroblasts. These give origin to olfactory nerve fibres which grow to the olfactory bulb of the cerebral hemisphere. In the same way fibres from the vomeronasal epithelium are growing to the accessory bulb. The external nose is formed during the facial development (see there).

The gustatory apparatus

From the cranial nerves VII, IX, X nerve fibres are growing into the tongue. They are connected to the taste buds inside the taste papillae.

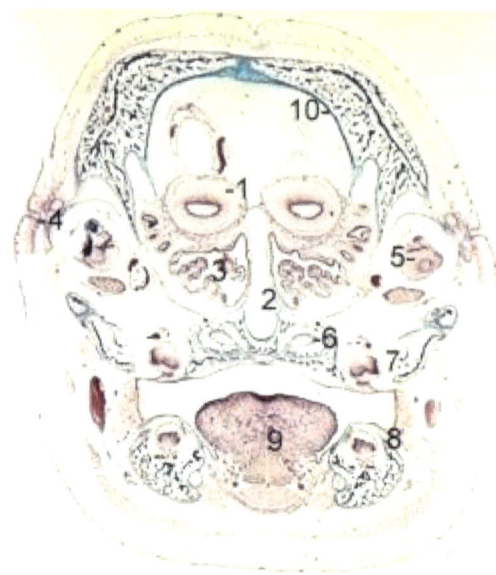

Fig.87: Pig embryo, 14 cm CRL, xtrichrome (from Künzel and Knospe, 1987): olfactory bulb (1), nasal septum (2), nasal conchae with olfactory epithelium (3), eye lids (4), ocular bulb (5), vomeronasal organ (6), maxilla with tooth germ (7), mandible with tooth germ (8), tongue (9), dura and frontal bone (10).

For somatic efferent nerves see the skin.

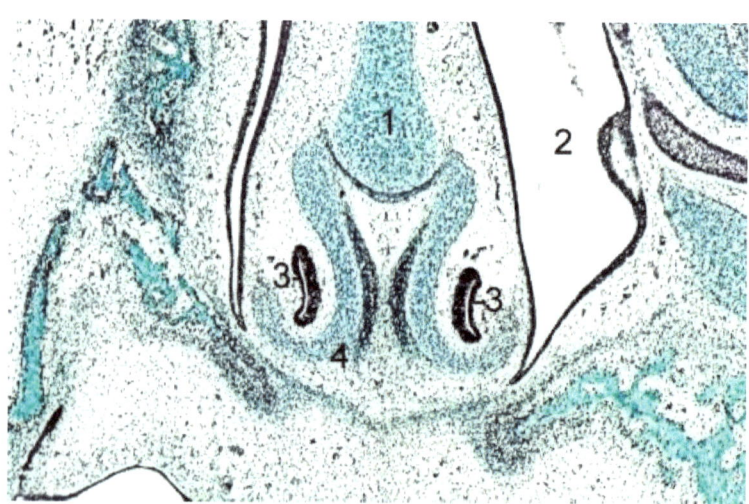

Fig. 88: Cat embryo, 34 days, cross section, xxtrichrome: nasal septum (1), nasal cavity (2), vomoronasal organ (3, Jacobson's organ), vomeronasal cartilage (4).

The Endocrine Organs

The Pineal Gland

A small ridge at the cranial neuropore, the optic torus, is reflected ventrally during the neurulation process forming the nervous part of the hypophysis. The adenohypophysis originates from the Rathke's pouch which appears in the roof of the stomatodaeum and extends in front of the buccopharyngeal membrane towards the optic torus.

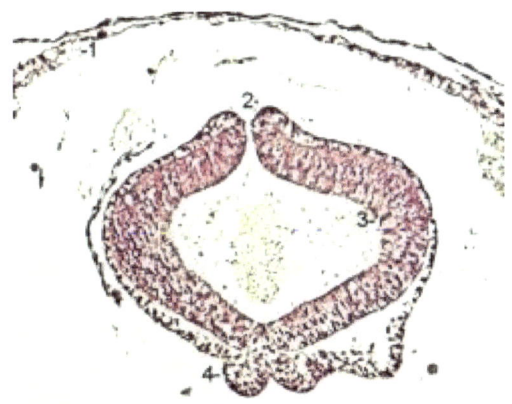

Fig.89: Chicken embryo, 18 h, cross section, xxHE: amniochorion (1), cranial neuropore (2), Prosencephalon (3), Torus opticus (4).

Fig.90: Cat embryo, 15 days, longitudinal section, xHE: diencephalon (1), optic torus (2), Rathke's pouch (3), stomatodaeum (4), primitive pharynx (5), pericardial swelling (6).

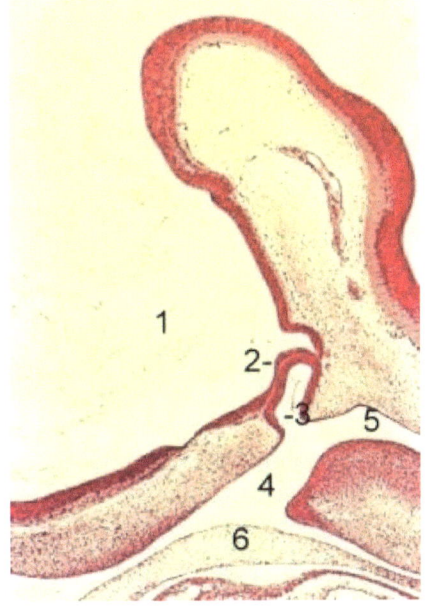

Very soon both rudiments are connected and proliferating. The Rathke's pouch transforms into a vesicle connected only by a small epithelial duct, the craniopharyngeal duct, to the pharyngeal roof until it loses later its attachment.

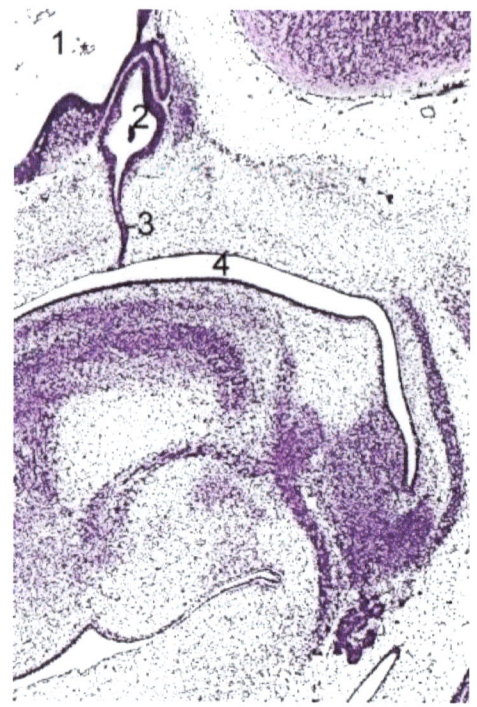

Fig.91: Cat embryo, 25 days, longitudinal section, x HE: diencephalon (1), Rathke's pouch (2), craniopharyngeal duct (3), primitive pharynx (4).

The median part of the former pouch is the pars intermedia with remnants of the lumen, the lateral part proliferates forming extensions round the diencephalic stalk and in this way the pars tuberalis and the pars anterior. During the fetal histogenesis all parts proliferate and differentiate. The remnant of the craniopharyngeal duct is visible up to day 37.

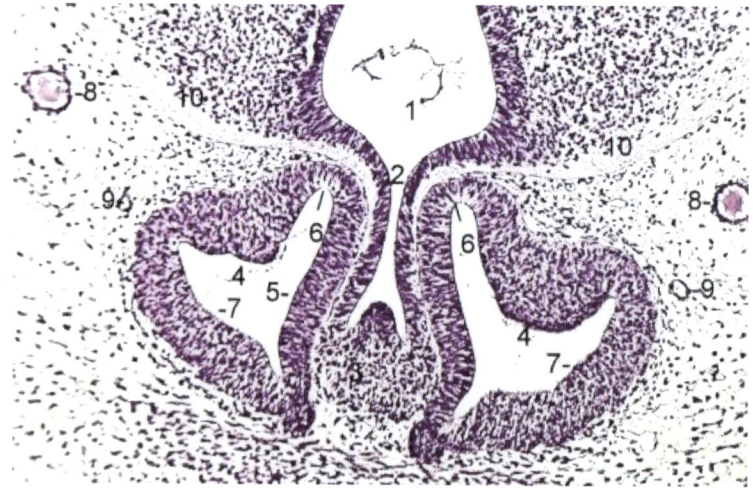

Fig.92: Cat embryo, 29 days, cross section, xxHE: Ventriculus tertius (1), Recessus infundibuli (2), Pars proximalis neurohypophysis (3), Cavum hypophysis (4), Pars intermedia adenohypophysis (5), Pars infundibularis (tuberalis) adenohypophysis (6), Pars distalis adenohypophysis (7), Circulus arteriosus cerebri (8), Plexus cavernosus (9), Hypothalamus (10)

Comparative Embryology

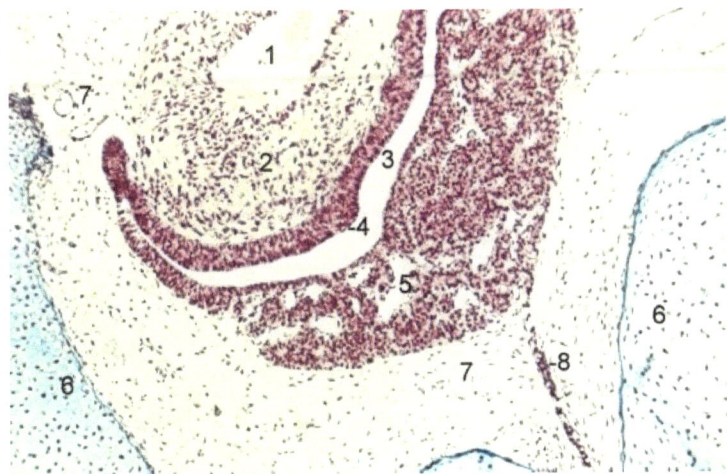

Fig.93: Cat embryo, 36 days, longitudinal section, xxtrichrome: Recessus infundibuli (1), Neurohypophysis (2), Cavum hypophysis (3), Pars intermedia (4), proliferating Pars distalis (5), Cartilago sphenoidalis (6), Plexus cavernosus (7), remnant of the Ductus craniopharyngeus (8).

The Adrenal Gland

The adrenal gland of higher vertebrates has two primordia, the mesodermal suprarenal cortex which develops from mesothelium between the mesentery and the gonad, and the ectodermal medulla which develops together with other paraganglia from sympathetic nerve cells of the neural crest.

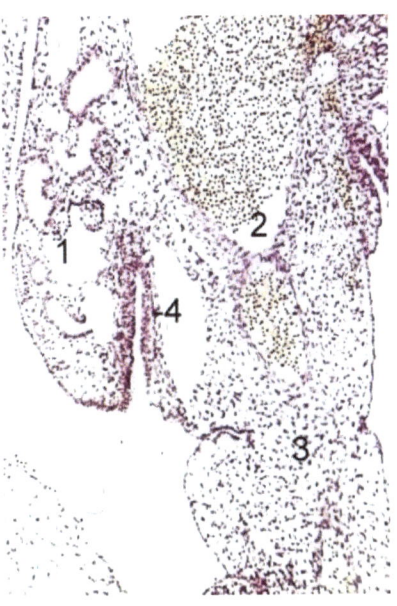

Fig.94: Cat embryo, 21 days, cross section, xxAzan: mesonephros (1), aorta (2), mesentery (3), suprarenal primordium (4).

With day 23 the mesothelial cells proliferate into cell cords inside the abdominal wall next to the aorta. After the ascensus of the metanephros, the suprarenal organs are in contact with the kidneys on both sides. The medulla cells invade from day 25 on the suprarenal organ from the hilus. Both parts proliferate, the cortex even in two different steps, but a clear zonation is not visible before birth. Therefore the fetal suprarenals are relatively large and already secreting. This is very important for the duration and regulation of the pregnancy. Shortly before birth the fetal cortex undergoes involution up to the first 3-4 weeks of life.

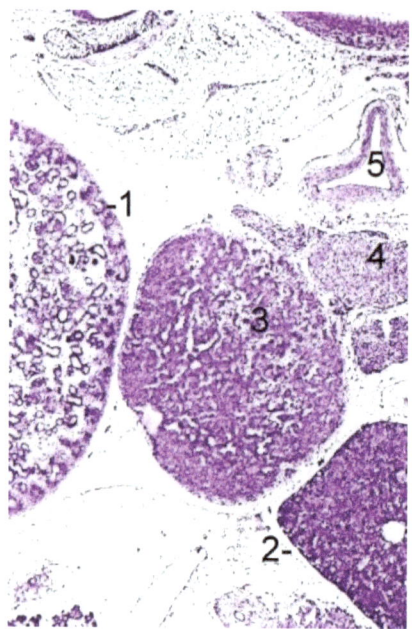

Fig.95: Cat embryo, 36 days, longitudinal section, xHE: metanephros (1), liver (2), proliferating suprarenal organ (3) in contact with the medulla (4), aorta (5).

Fig.96: Cat embryo, 55 days, cross section, xxHE: capsule (1), cortex still unzonated (2), medulla (3).

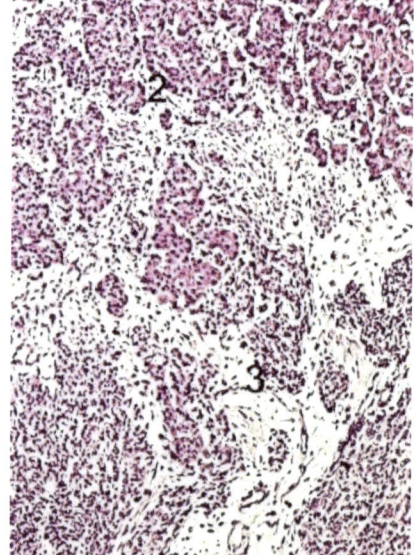

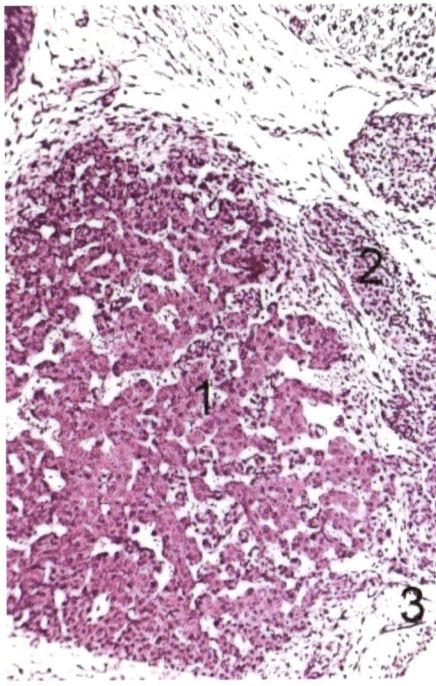

Fig.97: Suprarenal, Cat fetus 55 days, xxHE: epithelial strands of the cortex (1) and the medullary organ (2), capsule (3).

Fig.98: Suprarenal, Cat fetus, 58 days, xxHE: epithelium and capillaries (1) start the formation of the cortical zones, cell clusters (2) and ganglia cells are now representing the medulla.

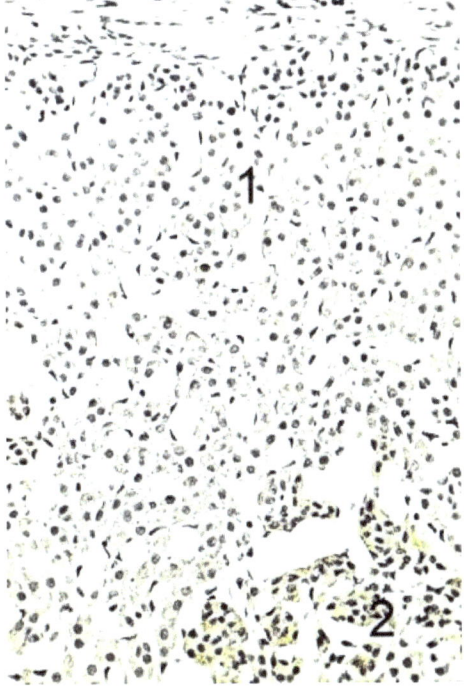

The Thyroid and the Parathyroid Glands

These glands are derivatives from pharyngeal pouches and the hypobranchial region (see primitive pharynx). All these glands originate from the endodermal epithelium of the primitive pharynx. The thyroid gland has a prolonged contact with the primitive pharynx in form of the thyreoglossal duct. Already with 14 days they form epithelial cords which proliferate into the branchial or hypobranchial mesenchyme. Thyroid and parathyroid gland get into contact by the growth of the esophagus and the trachea. About day 33 the parathyroid glands and the ultimobranchial body are incorporated into the thyroid gland. Already with 38 days the thyroid gland produces thyreoglobulin inside primitive follicles. The thymic cells of the dorsal recess of the third and fourth pouch are fast growing along the neck.

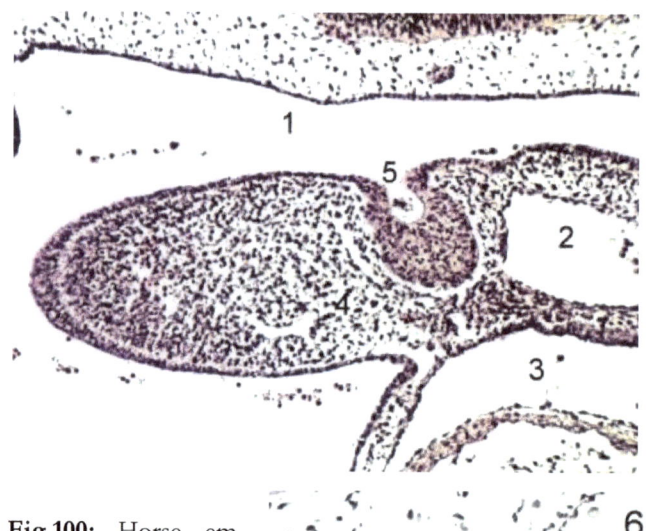

Fig.99: Cat embryo, 17 days, longitudinal section, xxHE: primitive pharynx (1), third aortic arch artery (2), pericardial cavity (3), first pharyngeal arch (4), thyroid pit (5).

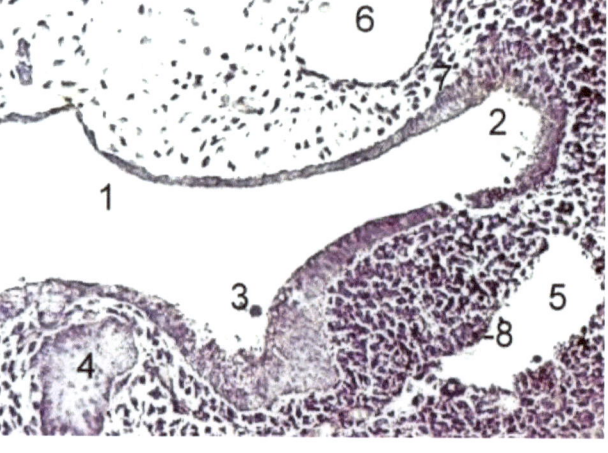

Fig.100: Horse embryo, 21 days, cross section, xxHE: primitive pharynx (1), dorsal recess of the third pharyngeal pouch (2), ventral recess of the third pharyngeal pouch (3), thyroid primordium (4), third aortic arch artery (5), dorsal aorta (6), thymic primordium (7), parathyroid primordium (8).

Comparative Embryology

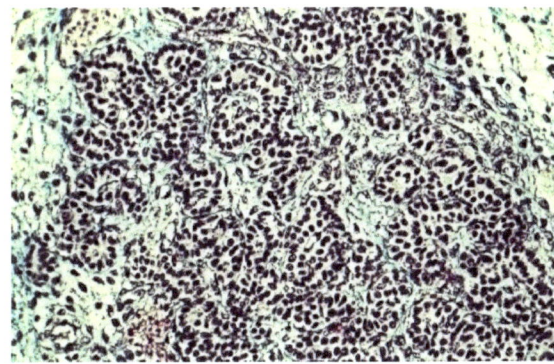

Fig.101: Cattle embryo, 22 cm CRL, xxtrichrome: parathyroid primordium with proliferating cell cords.

Fig.102: Cat embryo, 29 days, cross section, xxtrichrome: vertebral primordium (1), muscle blastema (2), esophagus (3), trachea (4), Ggl. nodosum (5), carotid (6), para-thyroid (7), thyroid (8).

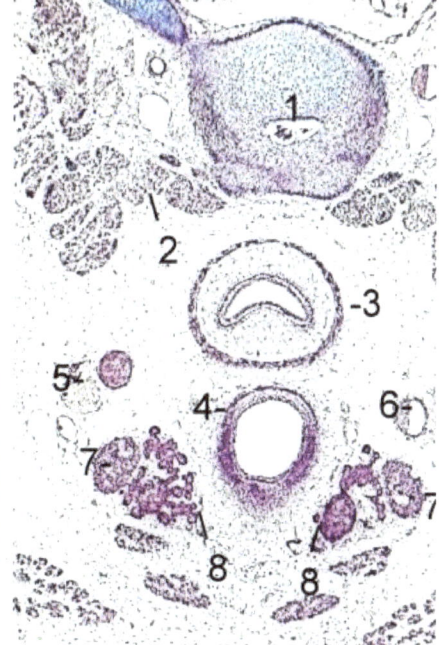

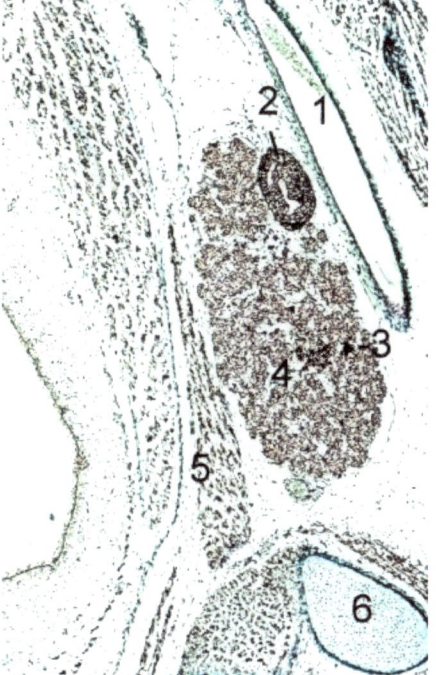

Fig.103: Cat embryo, 36 days, longitudinal section, xtrichrome: carotid (1), parathyroid (2), ultimobranchial body (3), thyroid (4) forming cell cords, long hyoid muscles (5), clavicle (6).

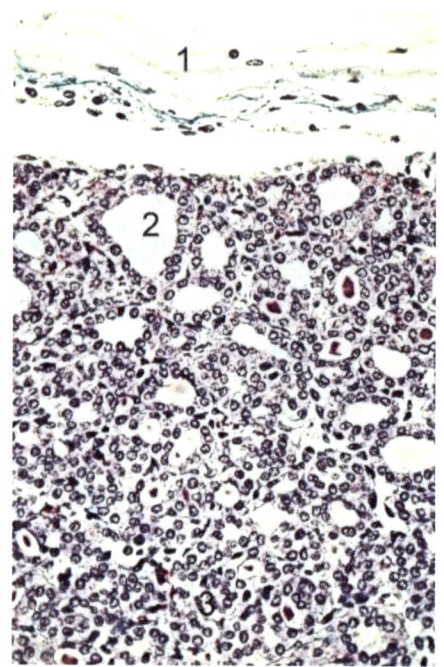

Fig.104: Sheep embryo, 17,5 cm CRL, cross section, xxtrichrome: Capsule (1), primitive follicles with thyreoglobolin (2), cell cords of parafollicular cells (3).

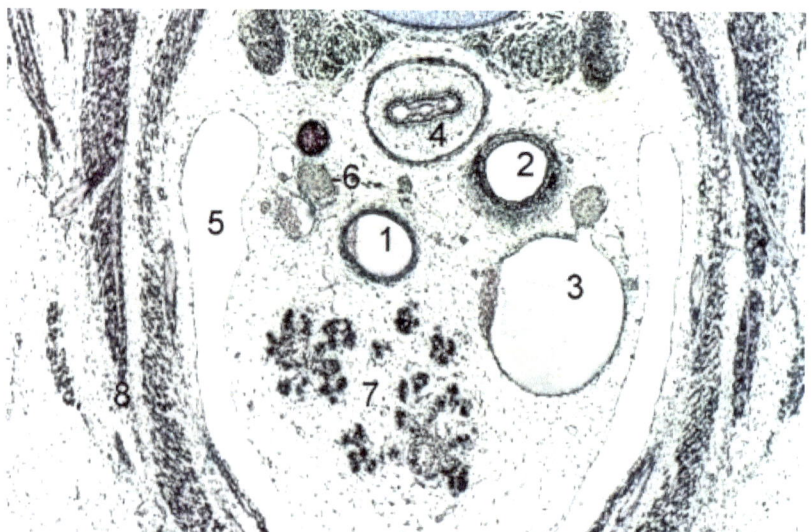

Fig.105: Cat embryo, 29 days, cross section, xtrichrome: brachiocephalic trunk (1), trachea (2), cranial caval vein (3), esophagus (4), pleural cavity (5), Ggl. nodosum n. vagi (6), thymus (7), intercostal muscles (8).

The Skin and its Derivatives

After the separation of the neural ectoderm the remaining ectoderm is forming the epidermis and all epidermal organs. Corium and hypodermis are mesodermal. The ectoderm consists initially of a single layer, but soon a second, superficial layer, called periderm (epitrichium), and additional layers are formed above a primitive basal membrane.

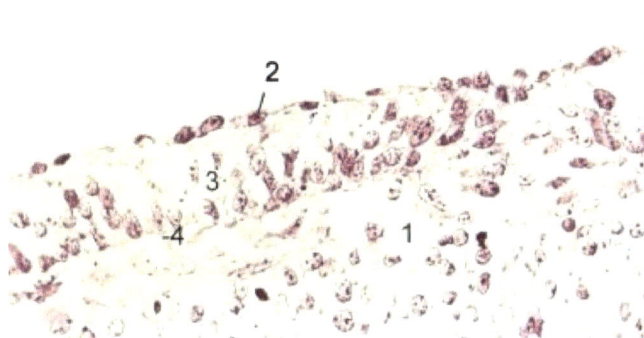

Fig.106: Cat embryo, 30 days, cross section, xHE: Corium (1), Periderm (2), layers of ectodermal epithelium (3), primitive basal membrane (4).

Fig.107: Cat embryo, 53 days, cross section, xxHE: hair germ (1), club-hair (2), sebaceous gland bud (3), sweat gland primordium (4), periderm (5).

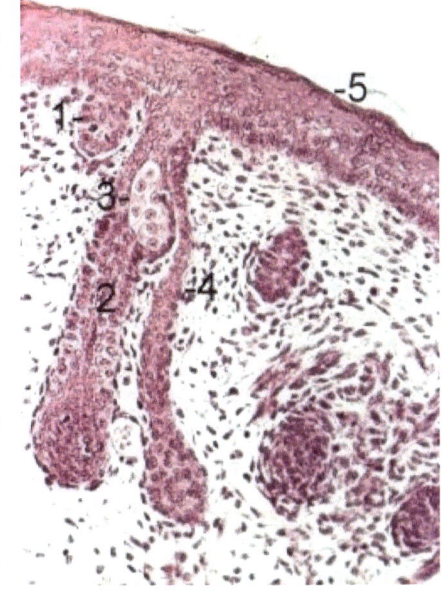

During the third trimester of the gestation the first hairs and glands develop from an epithelial downgrowth of the basal layer of the epidermis into the underlying dermis. Soon these hair germs become club-shaped with a sebaceous and a sweat gland primordium at their distal part. The first hairs are sinus hairs in the head region of the fetus. Soon a keratinized hair shaft is formed with peripherical cells as epithelial root sheat. The surrounding mesenchyme is condensed to the hair follicles.

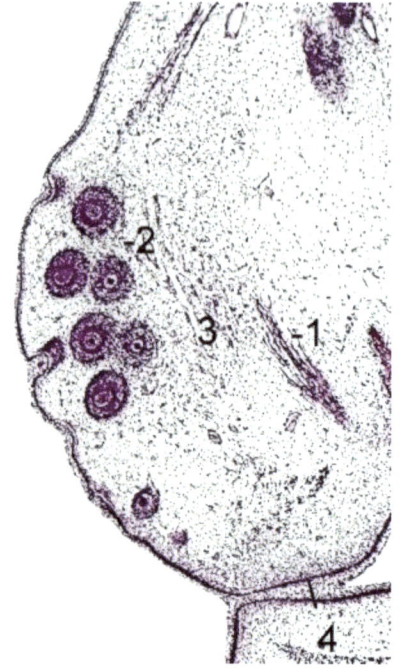

Fig.108: Cat embryo, 33 days, x trichrome: upper lid with muscle blastema (1), sinus hairs in development (2), larimal nerve (3), synechia of the lids (4).

Fig.109: Newborn cat, lip gland, xxtrichrome: activated sweat gland (1), sinus hair (2), sebaceous gland (3), blood vessel (4), cutaneous nerv (5), hairs shortly before their appearance (6).

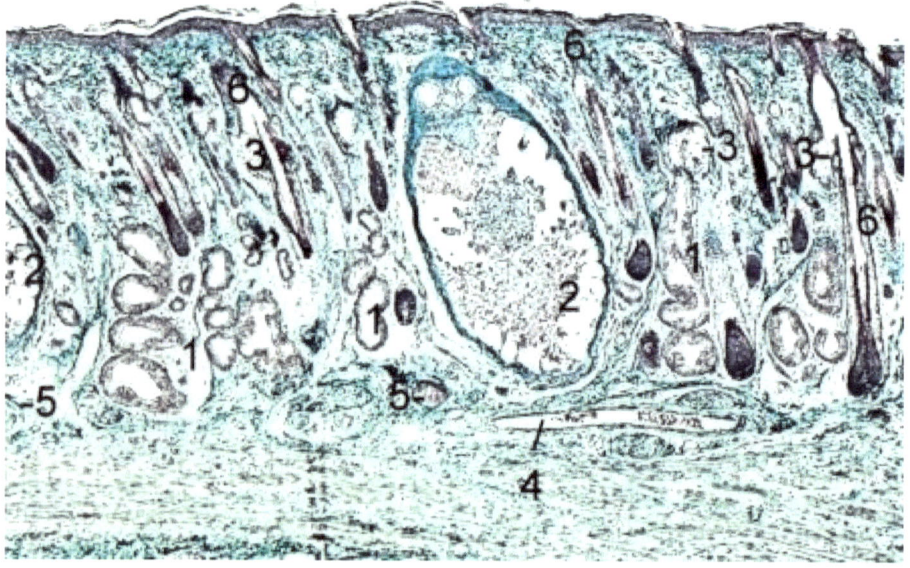

During the fetal histogenesis together with the hairs also skin nerves and their receptors develop. The upper lip of the cat, rich with sinus hairs, sebaceous gland and sweat gland, shows shortly before birth (58-62 days) a strong activity of the glands - the lip gland of the cat.

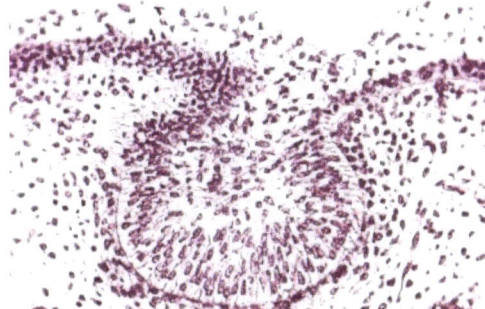

Fig.110: Mammary bud, sheep embryo, 3 cm CRL, cross section, xxHE.

Independent from hairs the sudoriferous glands and also the mammary gland arise as epidermal buds during the last trimester. The buds of the mammary gland grow along the mammary ridges or lines, linear thickenings of the epidermis, which appear already with 24 days. From these buds solid epidermal sprouts grow into underlying mesenchyme. In the last trimester the sprouts, the later lactiferous ducts, become canalized. In ruminants also the external part of the buds is growing to form the papillae.

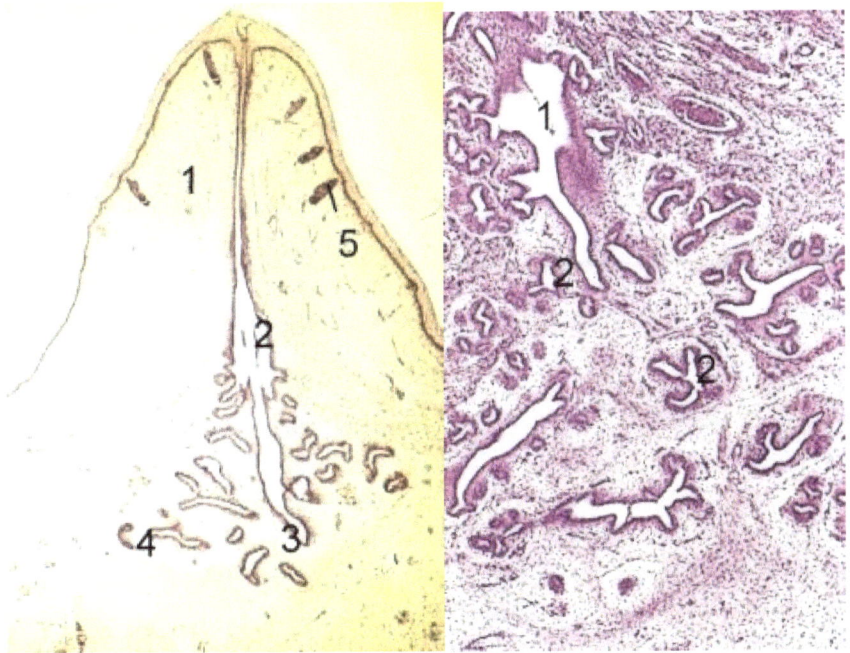

Fig. 111 (left side): sheep embryo, mammary gland, 20 cm CRL, xtrichrome: papilla (1), papillary duct and cisterna (2), canalized glandular ducts (3), solid sprouts.
Fig. 112 (right side): Cat, prenatal, xHE: Cistern (1) and glandular sprouts (2).

The sudoriferous glands begin to develop in the last trimester in the cat's footpads of the forelimbs and hindlimbs with their digital-, metacarpal-, metatarsal-, carpal- and tarsal pads and also the carpal glands.

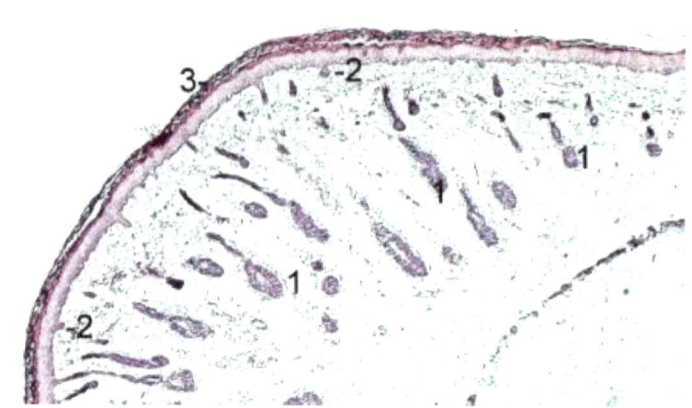

Fig.113: Cat embryo, 53 days, digital pad, xtrichrome: sudoriferous glands (1), gland buds as solid sprouts (2), the already keratinized epidermis (3).

Claws

Claws are local modifications of the skin. The epidermis is reflected, forming the unguicular crest during the second trimester. The underlying dermis is fusing with the periosteum. Later (during the third trimester) it develops the longitudinal interdigitations with the epidermal laminae. The lateral wall of the epidermis is compressed and early keratinized.

Fig.114: Cat embryo, 34 days, claw, xxtrichrome: cartilage of the distal (1) and middle (2) phalanges, phangeal joint (3), bone tip of the distal phalanx (4), future wall of the claw (5), digital pad (6), digital nerve (7), tendon of the extensory muscle (8).

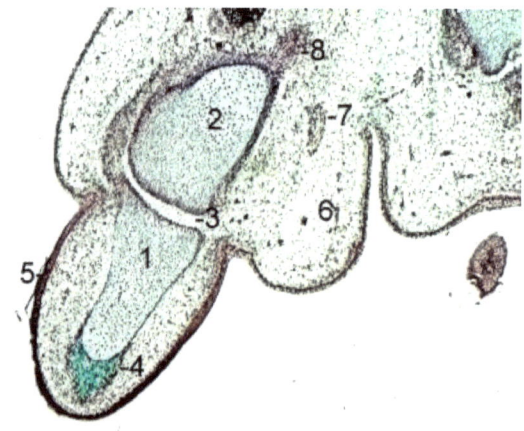

The Locomotive Apparatus

The Skeleton
The prenatal development is characterized by three main phases: the mesenchymal skeleton, already formed around day 11 with the notochord, later with somites (13 days), pharyngeal arches and limb buds (18 days). The cartilage skeleton arising during stage 14 (22 days), and the bony skeleton formed by intramembranous and endochondral ossification from stage 16/17 (26-30 days) on. The mesenchymal skeleton survives as periosteum in different ligaments, joint capsules, syndesmoses and intervertebral discs. The cartilage skeleton is reduced up to birth to the epiphyseal- and tympanic-cartilages, and survives as laryngeal, tracheal, joint, rib, sternal, nasal cartilages and synchondroses. In the newborn cat all primary centers are present, except the carpal and distal tarsal bones. The secondary and tertiary centers are formed postnatal from the first week on up to the second year.

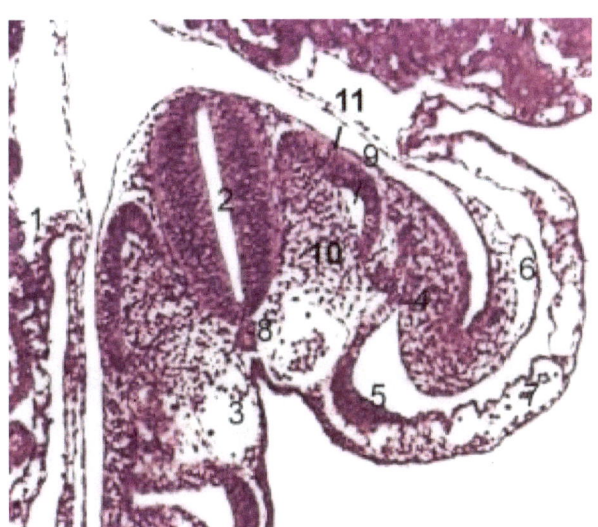

Fig.115: Cat embryo, 19 days, cross section, xxHE: Placenta (1), neural tube (2), aorta (3), somite stalk (4), mesothelium and coeloma (5), somatopleura (6), visceropleura (7), notochord (8), somatocoel (9), sclerotome (10), dermatomyotome (11).

The axial skeleton
The paraxial mesoderm is segmented forming the somites, which appear in cranial-caudal sequence. With 17 days they are transformed to an outer dermatomyotome and inner more scattered cells, the sclerotome. The cells of the sclerotomes migrate ventromedially to surround the neural tube and enclose the notochord. The caudal portion of each sclerotome unites with the cranial portion of the next. In this way they form the condensed intersegmental mesenchyme model of each vertebra. The cranial portion of the 1st cervical sclerotome unites with occipital sclerotomes. The notochord will later form the nucleus of the intervertebral discs.

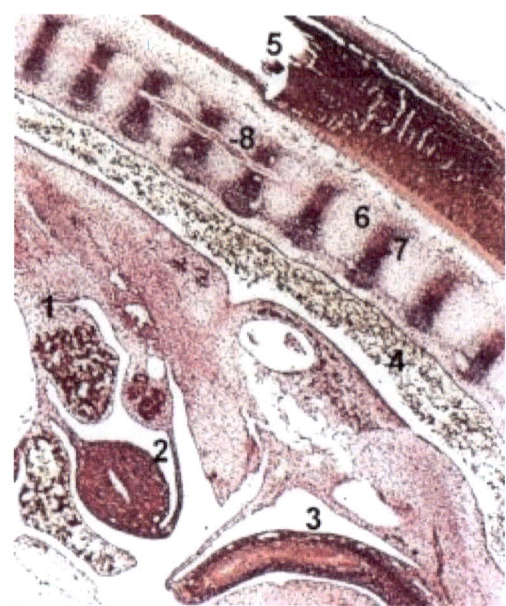

Fig.116: Cat embryo, 28 days, longitudinal section, xHE: liver (1), stomach (2), urogenital sinus and umbilical artery (3), aorta (4), neural tube (5), vertebral blastem (6), intervertebral disk (7), remnant of the notochord (8).

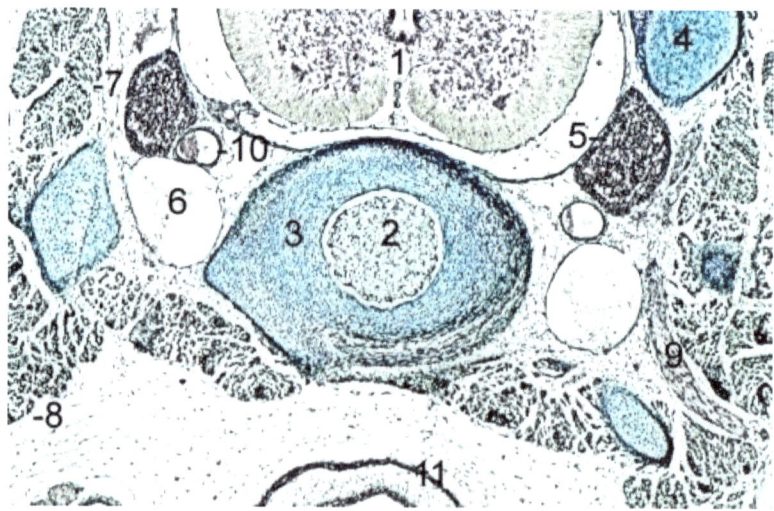

Fig.117: Cat embryo, 34 days, cross section, xxtrichrome: primitive spinal cord (1), remnant of the notochord (2), cartilaginous vertebral body (3), - and process (4), spinal ganglion (5), vertebral plexus (6), epaxial myoblasts (7), hypaxial myoblasts (8), spinal nerve (9), vertebral artery (10), esophagus (11).

Comparative Embryology

From stage 14 on the mesenchymal skeleton is transformed to cartilage. The vertebral arch is dorsally still open. Primary centers of ossification appear one for the body and one in each half of the neural arch from 26-30 days onwards. Ossification spreads but the individual centers remain separated by intervening cartilage. They fuse after birth. Ribs develop from mesenchymal extensions of the costal processes of the developing thoracic vertebrae by endochondral ossification. The sternebrae develop from bilateral mesenchymal bars. They ossify endochondrally from single centers.

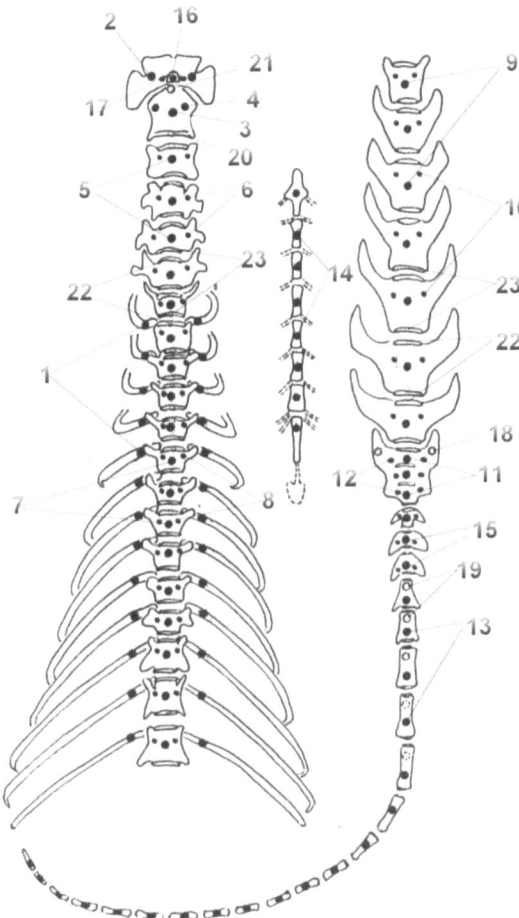

Fig.118: Ossification centers of the axial skeleton (from Knospe et al. 2004): stage 18 Costae I-XIII (1), Atlas, Arcus dorsalis incl. Alae (2), Axis, Corpus (3), Axis, Arcus (4), Vertebrae cervicales III-VII: Corpus (5), Arcus (6); Vertebrae thoracicae I-XIII: Corpus (7), Arcus (8); Vertebrae lumbales I-VII: Corpus (9), Arcus (10); Vertebrae sacrales I-III: Corpus (11), Arcus (12); stage 19 Vertebrae caudales I-XX (XXIII), Corpus (13), Sternebrae I-VIII (14), Vertebrae caudales I-VIII (X), Arcus (15); stage 20 Axis, Dens (16); stage 21 Atlas, Arcus ventralis (17), Vertebrae sacrales I, Pars lateralis (18); postnatally Vertebrae caudales IV-VI (VIII), Arcus haemales (19), Axis, Epiphysis caudalis (20), Axis, Apophysis versus Dens (21), Vertebrae cervicales (excl. Atlas, Axis), thoracicae, lumbales, sacrales, caudales: Epiphysis cranialis (22) und Epiphysis caudalis (23).

The anpendicular skeleton

The mesenchymal model of the skeleton is formed inside the limb buds in a complicated way influenced by different inducing factors like the apical ectodermal ridge, the polarizing zones and apoptotic processes. Already with 22 days the mesenchyme is transformed step by step to the cartilage model, visible even from the external view. Further growth of the cartilage model is achieved by interstitial growth of the cartilage and appositional growth from the perichondrium.

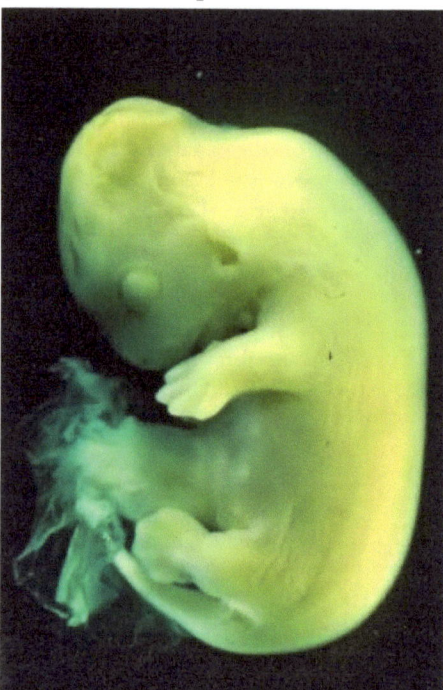

Fig.119: Cat embryo, 25 days with the cartilage model of all bones inside the limb buds.

From day 26 on the cartilage undergoes the process of endo- and perichondral ossification (for details see textbooks of histology). The time of appearance of primary centers varies according to species. In general however, they develop before midterm of gestation.

Fig.120(next page): Cat embryro, 44 days, longitudinal section of the forelimb, xtrichrome: scapula (1), epiphysis of the humerus (2), diaphysis of the humerus (3), blastema of the triceps muscle (4), future carpal joint (5), periosteal bone of the distal phalanx (6). **Fig.121:** Ossification of the forelimb of the cat (after Knospe et al. 2004): stage 17: Scapula (1), Clavicula (2), Diaphyses of Humerus (3), Radius (4) and Ulna (5), Ossa metacarpalia II-V (6), Phalanges distt. I-V (7); stage 18: Diaphysis of Os metacarpale I (8) and Phalanges proxx. II-V (9); stage 19: Diaphyses of Phalanx prox.I (10) and Phalanges mediae II-V (11); postnatal ossification (A): 1-2. week (LW) Caput humeri (12); 2.-3.LW Capitulum humeri (13), dist. Epiphyses of the Ossa metcarpalia II-V (14); 3.-4. LW Os carpi centrale (15), Os carpi accessorium (16), Ossa carpalia II-IV (17), Caput radii (18), Trochlea radii (19), Caput ulnae (20), prox. Epiphyses of Phalanges proxx. II-IV (21); 3.-5. LW Os carpi intermedium (22), Os carpale I (23), prox. Epiphyses of Phalanges mediae II-V (24); 4.-5. LW Trochlea humeri (25), prox. Epiphysis of Phalanx prox. V (26); 4.-6. LW Os carpi radiale (27), Os carpi ulnare (28), prox. Epiphysis of Os metacarpale I (29), prox. Epiphysis of Phalanx prox.I (30); 5.-6. LW Tuber olecrani (31);7.-9. LW Epicondylus medialis humeri (32); 7.-10. LW Epicondylus lateralis humeri (33); 7.-12. LW Proc. coracoideus (34), Tuberculum supraglenoidale (35); 9.-15. month (LM) Ossa sesamoidea proxx.II-V; 10.-16. LW Tuberculum minus humeri (36), 14.-26. LW Os sesamoideum musculi abductoris pollicis longi; 15.-22. LW Os sesamoideum prox. I; closure of metaphysis (B): 3.-7. LM Os carpi intermedioradiale (inkl. Os carpi centrale) (a); 4.-7. LM dist. Humerus (b); 5.-6.LM Apophysal plate of the scapula (c); 5.-7. LM prox. Radius (d); 6.-7. LM Apophysis of Os carpi accessorium (e); 6.-9. LM prox.

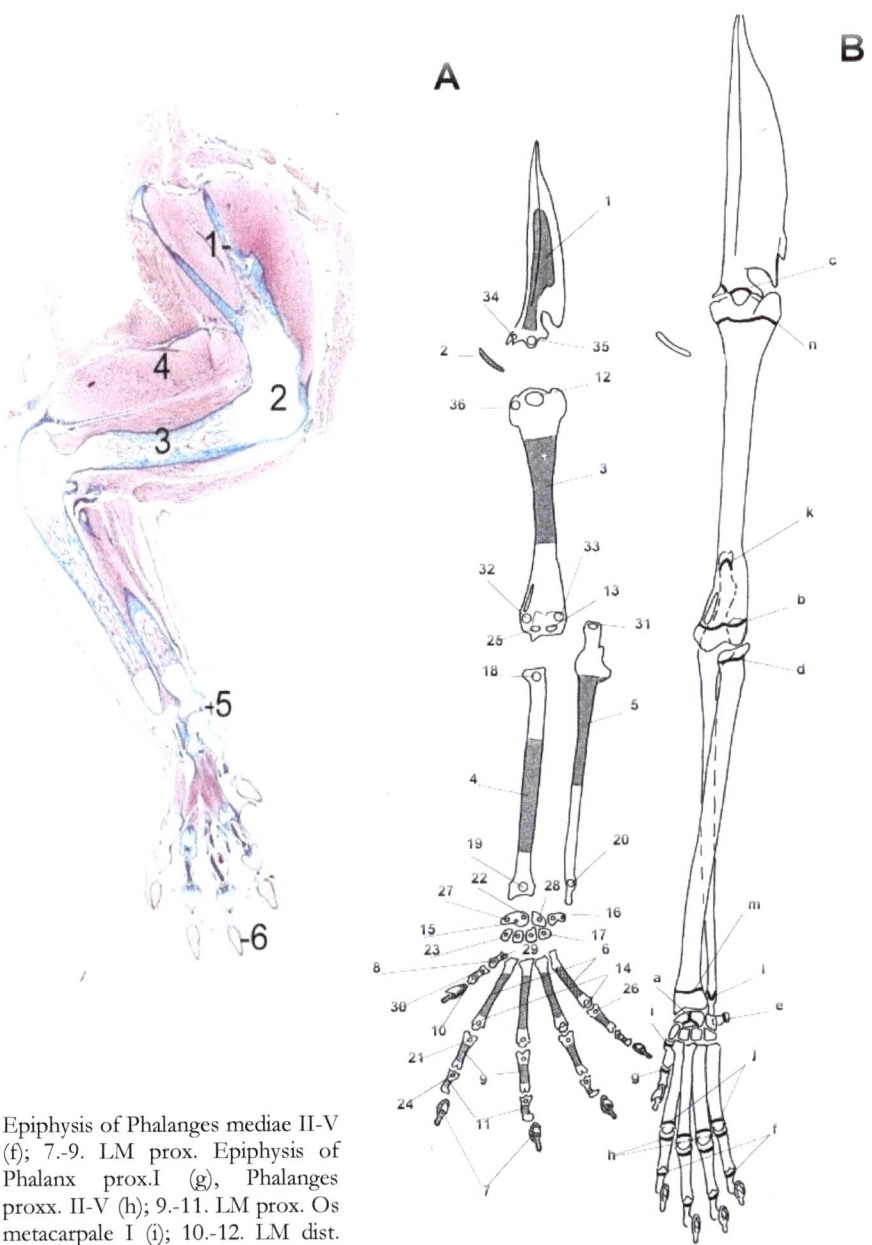

Epiphysis of Phalanges mediae II-V (f); 7.-9. LM prox. Epiphysis of Phalanx prox.I (g), Phalanges proxx. II-V (h); 9.-11. LM prox. Os metacarpale I (i); 10.-12. LM dist. Ossa metacarpalia II-V (j);12.-14. LM Tuber olecrani (k); 19.-22. LM dist. Ulna (l);19.-25. LM dist. Radius (m); 22.-24. LM prox. Humerus (n).

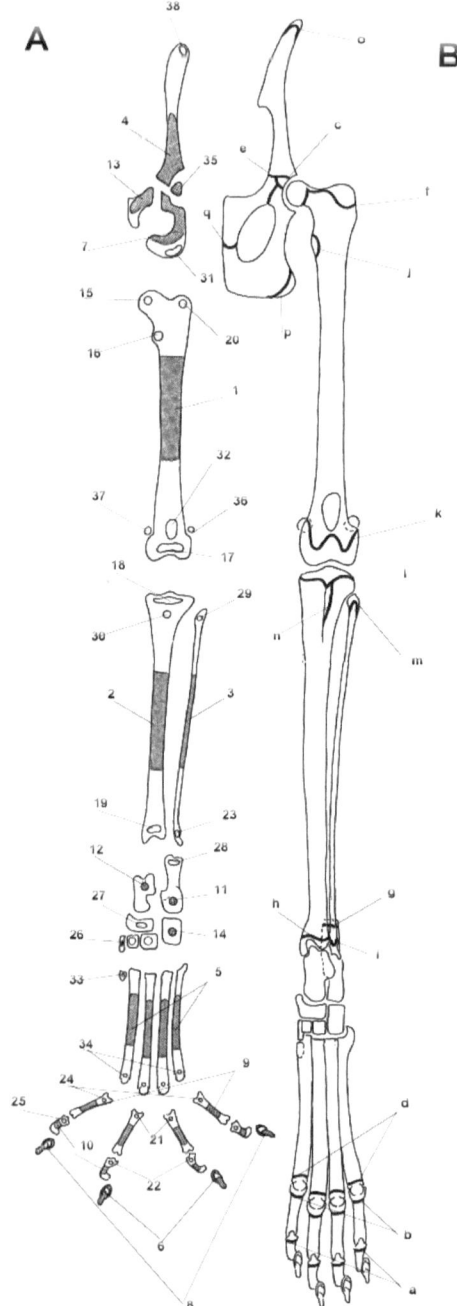

Fig.122: Ossification of the hind limb of the cat (after Knospe et al. 2004): stage 17 diaphysis of Os femoris (1), Tibia (2) & Fibula (3), Os ilium (4); stage 18 diaphysis of Ossa metatarsalia II-V (5), phalanges distt. III & IV (6); stage 19 Os ischii (7), phalanges distales II and V (8); stage 20 diaphysis of Phalanges proxx. II-V (9); stage 21 diaphysis of phalanges mediae II-V (10), Calcaneus (11), Talus (12), Os pubis (13), Os tarsale IV (14); **postnatal ossification (A):** 2.-3. LW Caput ossis femoris (15), Trochanter minor (16), Condylus ossis femoris (17), Condylus tibiae (18); 2.-4. LW Cochlea tibiae (19); 3.-4. LW Trochanter major (20), prox. Epiphysis of Phalanges proxx. III & IV (21) and mediae III & IV (22); 3.-5. LW Malleolus lateralis (23); 4.-5. LW prox. epiphysis of Phalanges proxx. II & V (24) und mediae II & V (25); 4.-6. LW Ossa tarsalia I-III (26), Os tarsi centrale (27); 5.-7. LW Tuber calcanei (28); 5.-8. LW Caput fibulae (29); 7.-10.LW Tuberositas tibiae (30);8.-11. LW Tuberculum ischiadicum (31); 8.-15. LW Patella (32);8.-16.LW Os metatarsale I (33), dist. epiphysis of Ossa metatarsalia II-V (34);9.-10. LW Os acetabuli (35); 12.-20. LW Os sesamoideum laterale musculi gastrocnemii (36); 20.-26. LW Os sesamoideum m. poplitei; 20.-26. LW Os sesamoideum mediale m. gastrocnemii (37); 26.-32. LW Crista iliaca (38); **ossification of epiphyseal cartilage (B):** 6.-8. LM prox. epiphysis of Phalanges mediae II-V (a); 7.-9. LM prox. epiphysis of Phalanges proxx. II-V (b); 8.-9. LM Os coxae, Area acetabuli (c); 10.-12. LM dist. epiphysis of Ossa metatarsalia II-V (d); 11.-12. LM epiphysis between Os ischii & Os ilium (e); 11.-14. LM Apophysis Caput ossis femoris & Epiphyse trochant. (f); 11.-15. LM Apophysis of Tuber calcanei (g); 12.-14. LM dist. epiphysis of Tibia (h) & Fibula (i); 12.-15. LM apophysis of Trochanter minor (j); 17.-20. LM epiphysis of Os femoris (k); 17.-21. LM prox. epiphysis of Tibia (l) & Fibula (m); 17.-22. LM apophysis of Tuberositas tibiae (n); 26. LM apophysis of Crista iliaca (o) & apophysis of Tuberculum isch. (p); epihyseal plate Oss. ischii/pubis (q).

The Skull

The mesenchymal model (desmocranium) is formed from mesodermal and mesectodermal material. The mesodermal material derived from occipital sclerotomes, the mesectodermal material derived from the neural crest via the pharyngeal arches. A chondral model for the later skull is found only at the base from a series of individual centres of chondrification, which merge to the chondrocranium. Later bones are formed by endochondral ossification. The sphenooccipital synchondrosis between basisphenoid and occipital bones is an important site for further growth in length of the base of skull. The bones of the vault of the cranium develop by intramembranous ossification of several individual centres. These enlarge by the development of spicules of bone arranged in a characteristically radiating pattern between

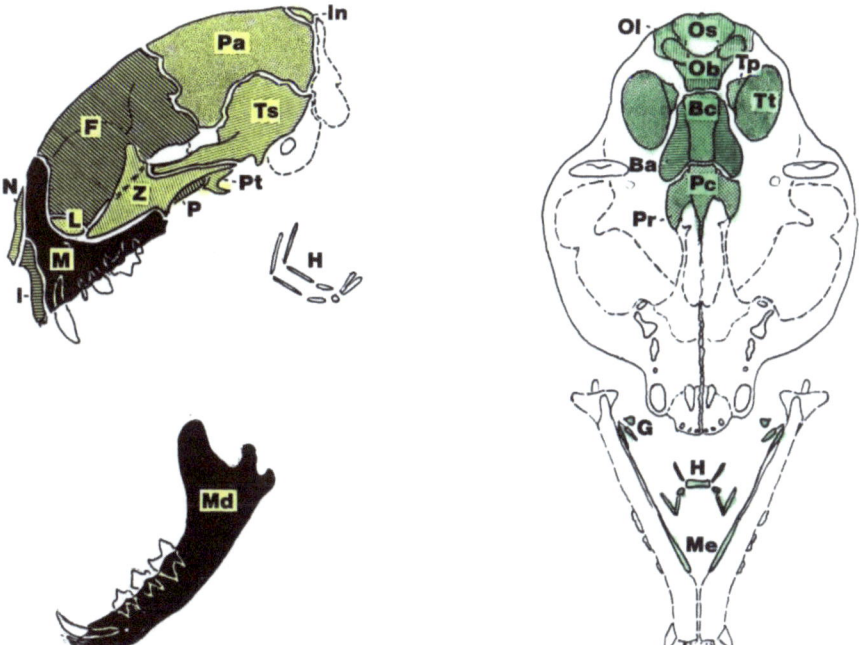

Fig.123: The ossification of the skull of the cat (after Knospe et al. 2004): stage 17 the maxilla (M) and mandibula (Md); stage 18 Os frontale (F), Os incisivum (I), Os palatinum (P), Os nasale (N), Os zygomaticum (Z), Os temporale, Pars squamosa (Ts), Os interparietale (In), Vomer, Os occipitale, Pars basilaris (Ob), Pars lateralis (Ol), Squama (Os), Ala basisphenoidalis (Ba), Os pterygoideum (Pt); stage 19 Os parietale (Pa), Os temporale, Pars tympanica (Tt), Ala presphenoidalis (Pr); stage 20 Os lacrimale (L), Corpus basisphenoidale (Bc), Corpus presphenoidale (Pc), Os temporale, Pars petrosa (Tp).

the sutures of the skull. At junctions between several bones larger areas of mesenchyme persist - the fontanelles. Postnatally the bones are remodelled to form inner and outer plates of compact bone separated by spongious bone, the diploe. The bones of the facial skeleton and the jaws develop by intramembranous and endochondral ossification forming the viscerocranium. The lower jaw region develops from the 1 st pharyngeal arch and the Meckel's cartilage. The symphysis of mandible fuses soon after birth in the horse and pig, whereas in the ruminants and carnivores the symphysis survive for a longer time. The hyoid bone develops from the cartilage of 2nd pharyngeal arch.

The Muscular System

Most of the muscles are of mesodermal origin. Exceptions are muscles of the head and myoepithelial cells which are ectodermal. Smooth muscles developing in various sites like the splanchnopleure. They retain the ability to divide. Cardiac muscles form mesoderm associated with the developing heart tube. Striated muscles develop from somites, lateral mesoderm or the pharyngeal arches. Soon after their initial appearance the somites are divided into 2 components: the sclerotome and dermatomyotome, which is subdivided into the dermatome - forming connective tissues of dermis, and the myotome - forming striated muscles. The cells of the sclerotome are scattered in cranial and caudal direction around the neural tube - forming the axial skeleton, but moved a half somite length cranially, whereas the myotome keep its position and is over bridging two skeletal segments.

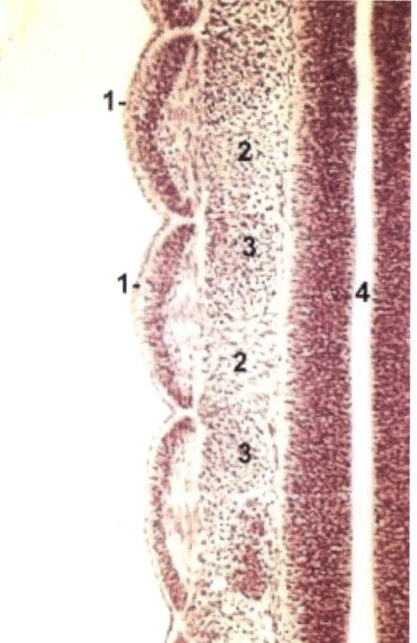

Fig. 124: Cat embryo, 17 days, horizontal section, xxHE: dermatomyotome (1), caudal parts (2), cranial parts of the sclerotomes (3) forming together the blastema of the vertebrates, neural tube (4).

With 17 days each myotome splits into a dorsal for the epaxial (Epimer) and a ventral division for the hypaxial (Hypomer) muscles innervated by the different branches of the spinal nerves. The mesoderm of the somatopleure

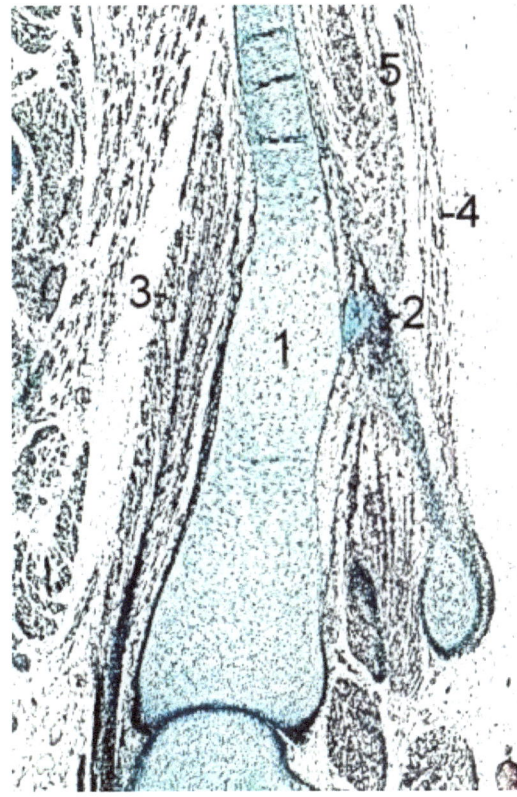

Fig. 125: Cat embryo, 31 days, cross section, xx trichrome: cartilage model of the scapula (1), desmal bone of the scapular spine (2), myoblastema of the subscapular muscle (3), myblastema of the deltoid muscle (4), myoblastema of the supraspinatus muscle (5),

gives rise to the thoracic and abdominal wall muscles. The limb buds are initially thickened outgrowths of the lateral mesoderm in which develop the limb musculature in mammals. The mesoderm of the pharyngeal arches give rise to the muscles of mastication, the facial muscles, the pharyngeal, the palatine and laryngeal muscles. The lingual muscles are hypobranchial. These muscular blastema consist of a particularly loose myoblasts, spindle shaped with centrally placed nuclei and presence of cytoplasmic myofilaments. Fusion of myoblasts leads to the formation of multinucleated myocytes or muscle fibres. The numbers of striated muscle fibres is achieved prenatally. Indeed the total numbers of fibres in a given muscle reduces significantly after birth. Tendons, ligaments, and synovial sheaths form independently from mesenchyme adjacent to developing muscles, linking up with them secondarily.

ClemensKnospe

References

Künzel, E. und Knospe, C.: Studienführer Embryologie. 5. ergänzte und erweiterte Auflage. Universitätsdruck FUB 1987.

Knospe, C.: Periods and Stages of the Prenatal Development of the Domestic Cat. Anat. Histol. Embryol. 31, 37-51 (2002).

Knospe, C., H. Roos und B. Vollmerhaus: Zur Entwicklung des Skeletts der Katze. Abstracts XXV. Congress of the European Association of Veterinary Anatomists, Oslo, July 2004.

ClemensKnospe

Index

A und I-Spermatogonien 9
A. centralis retinae 78
A. hyaloidea 78
A. mesenterica cranialis 26
A. pulmonalis 41
A. subclavia 40
A. vitellina 27
abraxas type 15
acardie 39,40
skelett 97
acoustic meatus 76
acrosomal enzymes 20
acrosomal phase 11
acrosomal vesicle 11
adamantoblasts 51
adenohypophysis 79
adrenal gland 81
adrenal medulla 73
Akrosomenkappe 11
akrosomal reaction 17
alar lamina 71
allantoamnion 28, 30
Allantochorion 28, 30
allantoic diverticulum 28
allantoid vessels 28
Allantois 26, 28, 32, 55
incus 81
ameloblasts 50
amniochorion 28
amnion 28
amphimixis 18
ampulla 67
anal atresia 55
anal membrane 55
anaphase 14
anisolecithal 16
anorectal canal 55
anovulatory 16
antiakrosin 15
Anti-Mullererian-factor 69
Antrum 12
aortic arch 41
aqueous chamber 74
arch arteries 47
archencephalon 70
areolae 33
artificial insemination 20
arytenoid swellings 47
ascensus of the kidneys 81
atretic follicles 15
atria 38
atrioventricular canal 39
atrioventricular ostium 39
atrioventricular sulcus 38
auditory meatus 48
auricular hillocks 48
auricular hillocks 76
autosomes 15
aveolar stage 60
axial mesoderm 26
azygos veins 42
basal lamina 71
blastocoele 23
blastocyst 23
blastoderm 25
blastogenesis 22
blastomeres 22
blastomerula 22
Blood vessels 36
bony skeleton 91
branchial nerves 47
brain vesicle 48,70
branchial arteries 38, 41
branchial cartilage 47
bronchial tree 58
bucconasal membrane 56
buccopharyngeal membrane 28, 45
bulbourethral gland 67
bulbus cordis 38
canalicular stage 60
cap phase 11
capacitation 20
Cardiac muscles 100
cardinal vein 38
cardinal veins 37,41
cardiogenic area 37
cartilage growths 94
cartilage skeleton 91
cartilages 91
caruncles 32
cauda equina 71
cavernose bodies 70
cementum 50
centers of ossification 93
cervical flexure 48, 71
cervical sinus 45
cervical sinus 48
chiasmata 11
choana 56
chondrocranium 98

chorioallantoic placenta 32
chorioallantoic vessels 30
chorion 30
chorion frondosum 32
chorionic gonadotropin 34
choriovitelline 32
choriovitelline placenta 29
choroid 74
choroid plexus 73
choroidal fissure 74
chromatids 11
ciliary body 74
ciliary body 75
circulatory changes during birth 42
classification of the placenta 32
claws 90
cleavage 21, 22
cloaca 55, 64
cloacal membrane 25, 55
closing membranes 46
cochlear pouch 77
coelom 26
coloboma 74
conception 23
conception hillock 21
conducting system 40
congenital cystic kidney 65
conjugation 23
conjunctiva 77
copula 46
corium 87
cornea 74
corona radiata 16
corona radiata 20
coronary sinus 39
corpus luteum 16
cortex 73
cortical cords 67
cortical vesicles 21
cotyledonary placenta 32
cranial nerves 74
craniopharyngeal duct 79
crossing over 11
crown-rump length 28
Cryptorchidism 70
Cytokinesis 14
cytokinesis 15
decidua 32, 34
deciduate placenta 32
deferent duct 67
dental buds 49
dental cuticle 50
dental laminae 49

dental papilla 50
dermatome 100
dermatomyotome 91
desmocranium 98
deuterencephalon 70
diakinesis 11
dictyotene 15
dictyotene stage 68
diencephalic vesicle 71
diffuse placenta 34
digestive system 45
dioestrous 16
diplotaen stage 11
diplotene stage 15
discoid placenta 32
dorsal and ventral plates 71
dorsal aorta 41
Drosophila type 15
duct of Arantii 41
duct of Botalli 43
duct of Cuvier 41
ductus arteriosus 41
duration of oestrous 16
dysphagia 41
ear 74
early development 22
ectoblast 24
ectopia cordis 40
ectopic implantation 29
efferent ductules 67
egg cell sizes 16
egg cells type 22
eggs 16
Eisenmenger syndrom 41
ejaculation 20
ejaculatory duct 67
embryo transfer 24
embryoblast 23
embryonal period 28
embryonic disc 23
embryotrophe 33
enamel epithelium 50
enamel prisms 50
Endocardial cushions 39
endocardial ridges 39
endocardial tubes 37
endochondral ossification 91
endocrine cells 73
endocrine organs 79
endoderm 24
endorphine 15
endothelial cells 36
endotheliochorial placenta 32

epididymal duct 67
epigenesis 24
epiglottal swellings 47
epimer 100
epiphyseal-cartilages 91
epiploic foramen 52
epithelial root sheath 50
epitheliochorial placenta 32
epitrichium 87
equal cleavage 22
esophagus 52
esophagus 57
external ear 76
extraembryonic membranes 23, 28
extraembryonic mesoderm 25
eye 74
eyelids 74, 75
face 48
facial clefts 48
facial muscles 100
female duct system 68
female gamete 15
fertilization 15, 20
fertilization membrane 21
fetal period 35
fetal suprarenals 82
fetogenesis 35
flagellum 11
follicles 15
folliculogenesis 15
folliculogenesis 68
fontanelles 99
foramen caecum 47
foramen ovale 39, 43
fore-, mid- and hindgut 28
forebrain 71
foregut 45
freemartin 70
frontonasal prominence 48
Gametes 15
Gametogenesis 9
ganglia 72, 74
gastric glands 52
gastric pits 52
gastrolienal ligament 52
gastrulation 24
gene manipulation 20
genital ridge 61
genital ridges 65
genital swellings 69
genital system 61
genital tubercle 69
germ layers 24

glioblasts 71
golgi phase 11
gonadocrinin 15
gonads 65
Graafian follicles 16,v20
gray matter 72
gustatory apparatus 77
gut 45
hair follicles 88
hair germs 87
hair shaft 89
hairs 87
hare-lip 56
hatching 23
head 48
heart 36
heart descend 38
heart loop 38
heart malformations 40
heart tube 37
heifer 70
hematomes 33
hematopoiesis 43
hematopoietic clusters 43
hemochorial placenta 32
hemocytoblasts 36
hemotrophe 33
hepatolienal period 43
hermaphrodits 70
heterosomes 15
hindbrain 48
hindbrain 71
hindgut 55
histiotrophe 33
histogenesis 35
holoblastic type 22
holonephros 61
homologous chromosomes 11
hyaloid artery 74
hyaloid substance 74
HY-antigen 23
hydrocephalus 73
hymen 69
hyoid arch 45
hypobranchial eminence 46
hypobranchial plate 46
hypobranchial region 84
hypodermis 87
hypomer 100
iliac arteries 41
impar tubercle 46
implantation 28
impregnation 20

incus 76
infracardial bursa 60
inhibin 15
inner glomerula 62
insemination 20
intermediate mesoderm 26
internal ear 77
interoestrous phase 16
interstitial cells 66
interventricular septum 39
intervertebral discs 91
intestinal portals 28, 45
intestinal rotation 55
intestines 54
intramembranous ossification 91
invitro-fertilization 24
iris 74
isolecithal 16
joint capsules 91
jugular veins 42
junctional zones 33
kidney ascend 63
labyrinthine placenta 32
lacrimal glands 75
lactiferous ducts 89
laryngeal muscles 100
laryngotracheal groove 57
larynx 46
larynx 57
lateral lingual swellings 46
lateral plate mesoderm 26
lateral plates 71
lens placode 74
leptotene stage 11
ligaments 93
ligaments 101
ligamentum arteriosum 41
limb buds 91
limb musculature 100
lingual muscles 100
lip gland 89
liver 45, 56
lower lip 48
lung 45
lung buds 58
lungs 57
lymph vessel 44
lymphatic sacs 44
lymphnodes 44
macrolecithal 16
macromeres 24
male duct system 66
malleus 76

mammary gland 89
mammary ridges 89
mandibular 48
mandibular process 45
mantle zone 71
marginal zone 71
mating 20
maturation phase 11
maxilla 48
maxillary process 45
Meckel's cartilage 47
Meckel's diverticulum 55
mediastinal cavity 60
mediastinum 60
medullary ascend 73
medullary cords 66
medullary period 43
megaloblastic period 43
meiosis 15
meiosis 9
meiosis 11
meiotic division 21
melanocytes 73
meroblastic type 22
merogony 22
mesectoderm 72
mesectoderm 98
mesectodermal mesenchyme 45
mesencephalon 71
mesenchymal skeleton 91
mesoderm 24
mesodermal plate 25
mesogastrium 52
mesolecithial 16
mesonephric duct 62
mesonephric fold 62
mesonephric ridge 62
mesonephros 62
mesothelial cells 81
metanephric blastem 62
metanephros 62
metaphase 11
metencephalic part 71
microlecithal 16
micromeres 24
midbrain 71
midbrain flexure 71
midgut loop 54
monoestrous 16
morphogenesis 24
morula 22
morulation 22
mosaic eggs 24

mucous cells 52
muellerian inhibiting factor 67
Mullerian duct 67
muscle fibres 100
muscles 100
muscles of mastication 100
myelencephalic part 71
myoblasts 100
myocytes 100
myotome 100
nasal cavity 77
nasal pit 56
nasal process 48
nasolacrimal duct 48
neck 48
neozonae 16
nephrogenic corpuscles 62
nephrogenic ridge 61
nephrostoma 61
nephrotomes 61
nervous System 70
neural crest 26
neural crests 70
neural crests 72
neural folds 26
neural plate 26
neural tube 70
neuroblasts 71
neuroepithelium 71
neuropore 70
neuropores 26
neurulation 26
non ascent of kidneys 63
nondeciduate placenta 32
notochord 25, 26, 91
occipital sclerotomes 98
odontoblasts 50, 73
oestrous 16
oestrous cycle 16
oestrous phases 16
olfactory bulb 77
olfactory nerve 77
olfactory pits 77
olfactory placodes 77
oligolecithal 16
omasum 53
omental bursa 52
omphalomesenteric artery 41
omphalomesenteric veins 37, 38
omphalopleure 29
oocytolemm 20
oogenesis 9, 15
oogonia 15, 68

operculum 45
optic cup 48, 74
optic stalk 74
optic torus 79
optic vesicle 74
oral cavity 56
organogenesis 28, 34
ossification centers 91
ostium primum 39
otic placode 74
otic vesicle 74
otocyst 77
outer glomerulum 61
ovarian cycle 16
oviduct 23
ovulation 15, 16, 20
ovum 15
oxyntic cells 52
oxytocin 15
palatal processes 56
palatine muscles 100
pancreas 45, 56
pancreatic diverticles 56
paraganglia 81
paragenital appendix 67
paramesonephric ducts 67
paranasal sinuses 57
paranephric ducts 68
paraplacenta 33
parathyroid glands 84
paraxial mesoderm 26
parietal flexure 48
Parthenogenesis 22
partial cleavage 22
parturition 15, 32
pelvic part 64
pericard 28
pericardial cavity 37, 60
perichondral ossification 94
perichondrium 94
periderm 87
peridontal membrane 50
perineum 55
periosteum 91
peritoneal cavity 60
perivitelline space 21, 22
persistent ductus arteriosus 40
persistent right aortic arch 40
PGC 65
phallic part 64
phallic tubercle 70
pharyngeal arches 38, 45, 98
pharyngeal clefts 46

pharyngeal muscles 100
pharyngeal pouch derivatives 47
pharyngeal pouches 46
pharyngeal pouches 84
physiological herniation 54
pineal gland 79
placenta 23, 28, 30
placental lactogen 34
placentation 30
placentomes 32
placodes 27, 48, 74
pleural cavities 60
pleural cavity 58
pleuropericardial septum 60
pneumato-enteric recesses 60
polar bodies 15
 polylecithal 16
polyoestrous 16
polyspermy 21
pontine flexura 48, 71
portal vein 42
postcytokinesis 12
postoestrous 16
postspermiation 13
prechordal plate 27
precytokinesis 16
predentine 50
preformation 24
pregnancy 20
preleptotene 11
preova 16
prepuce 70
preputial diverticle 67
prespermiation 12
primary bronchi 58
primary follicles 15
primary oocytes 15
primary palate 56
primary septum 37
primary spermatocytes 11
primitive follicles 84
primitive gut 26
primitive heart 37
primitive meninges 73
primitive node s. Hensen's node 24
primitive organs 26, 28
primitive pharynx 28, 45, 84
primitive streak 24
primordial follicles 15
primordial germ cells 9, 15
pronephric duct 61
pronephros 61
prooestrous 16

prophase 11
prosencephalon 71
prospective potency 24
prostate gland 67
protenor type 15
provoced ovulation 16
pseudoglandular stage 58
pulmonary arteries 41
pulmonic stenosis 41
pyloric stenosis 53
raphe 70
Rathke's pouch 79
reduplication 21
regulation eggs 24
Reichert's cartilage 47
renal agenesis 63
respiratory distress syndrome 60
respiratory system 56
retarded implantation 29
rete 67
reticulum 53
retina 74
rhombencephalon 71
ribs 93
rumen 53
salivary glands 49, 50
satellite cells 73
Schwann cells 73
sclera 74
sclerotome 71
sebaceous glands 87
second septum 39
secondary chorion 30
secondary oocytes 15
secondary palate 56
secundary follicles 16
segmental arteries 41
semicircular ducts 77
seminal epithelium 12
septum transversum 28
septum transversum 38
sex cords 66
sinovaginal bud 69
sinovaginal plate 69
sinus 38
sinus hairs 89
sinus venosus 40
situs inversus 40
skin and derivatives 87
skin glands 87
skin nerves 89
skin receptors 89
skull 98

smooth muscles 100
somatic pleura 26
somatopleura 26
somite stalk 26
somite stalk 61
somites 26
somites 91
sperm cells 16
spermatids 9, 11
spermatocytes 9
spermatocytogenesis 9, 10
spermatogenesis 9
spermatogonia 9
spermatogonia 9, 10
spermatozoa 16, 20
spermiation 13
spermiogenesis 9
spinal nerves 74
splanchnic pleura 26
spleen 44
stapes 76
stellate reticulum 50
sternebrae 93
stomach 45, 52
stomach rotation 52, 54
stomatodeum 45
striated muscles 100
subaortic stenosis 41
subcardinal veins 41
subclavian artery 41
subgerminal cavity 24
sudoriferous glands 89
sudoriferous glands 90
sulcus limitans 71
superfecundation 22
superfetation 22
supracardinal veins 41
suprarenal cortex 81
suprarenal organs 81
surfactant 60
sweat glands 87
synchondroses 91
syncytial trophoblast 24
syndesmochorial placenta 32
syndesmoses 91
synovial sheaths 101
taste buds 77
TDF 66
teeth develop 49
telencephalic vesicles 71
telolecithal 16
telophase 11
tendons 101

tertiary follicles 15
tertiary follicles 16
testibumin 15
tetrads 11
Tetralogy of Fallot 41
cardiovascular system 36
locomotor apparatus 91
skeleton 91
theriogenology 20
thymic cells 84
thyreoglobulin 84
thyreoglossal duct 46,84
thyroid 84
thyroid gland 46
thyroid placode 46
thyroid vesicle 46
tongue 46
trachea 57
tracheaesophageal septum 57
tracheoesophageal fistula 57
transferring 15
transitory organs 34
transitory structures 27
trophoblast 23
truncus arteriosus 38, 41
tubulus stage 11
twinning 21
tympanic membrane 76
ultimobranchial body 84
umbilical arteries 41
umbilical cord 34
umbilical stalk 28
umbilical veins 38, 41
umbilical vessels 30
unguicular crest 90
upper lip 48
urachus 55
urachus 64
ureter 64
ureteric bud 62
urethra 64
urethral folds 70
urethral groove 70
urinary bladder 64
urinary system 61
urogenital artery 41
urogenital fold 66
urogenital membrane 55
urogenital sinus 55, 64
urorectal septum 55, 64
uterine cycle 17
uterine horns 68
uterine tube 68

vaginal cycle 19
vaginal vestibule 69
valves 40
vasopressin 15
veins 41
vena cava 42
venous duct 41
ventricles 38
ventriculobulbic sulcus 39
vertebral column 91
vesical part 64
vesicular gland 67
vestibular pouch 77
vestibulum bursae 52
viscerocranium 99
visceropleura 26
vitelline arteries 34
vitellointestinal duct 28
Vv. hepaticae advehentes 41
Vv. hepaticae revehentes 41
Wharton's jelly 32
white matter 72
Wolffian duct 62
yolk 16
yolk platelets 22
yolk sac 26, 29, 36
zona 23
zona pellucida 16, 20
zonary placenta 32
zygote 15
zygotene stage 11

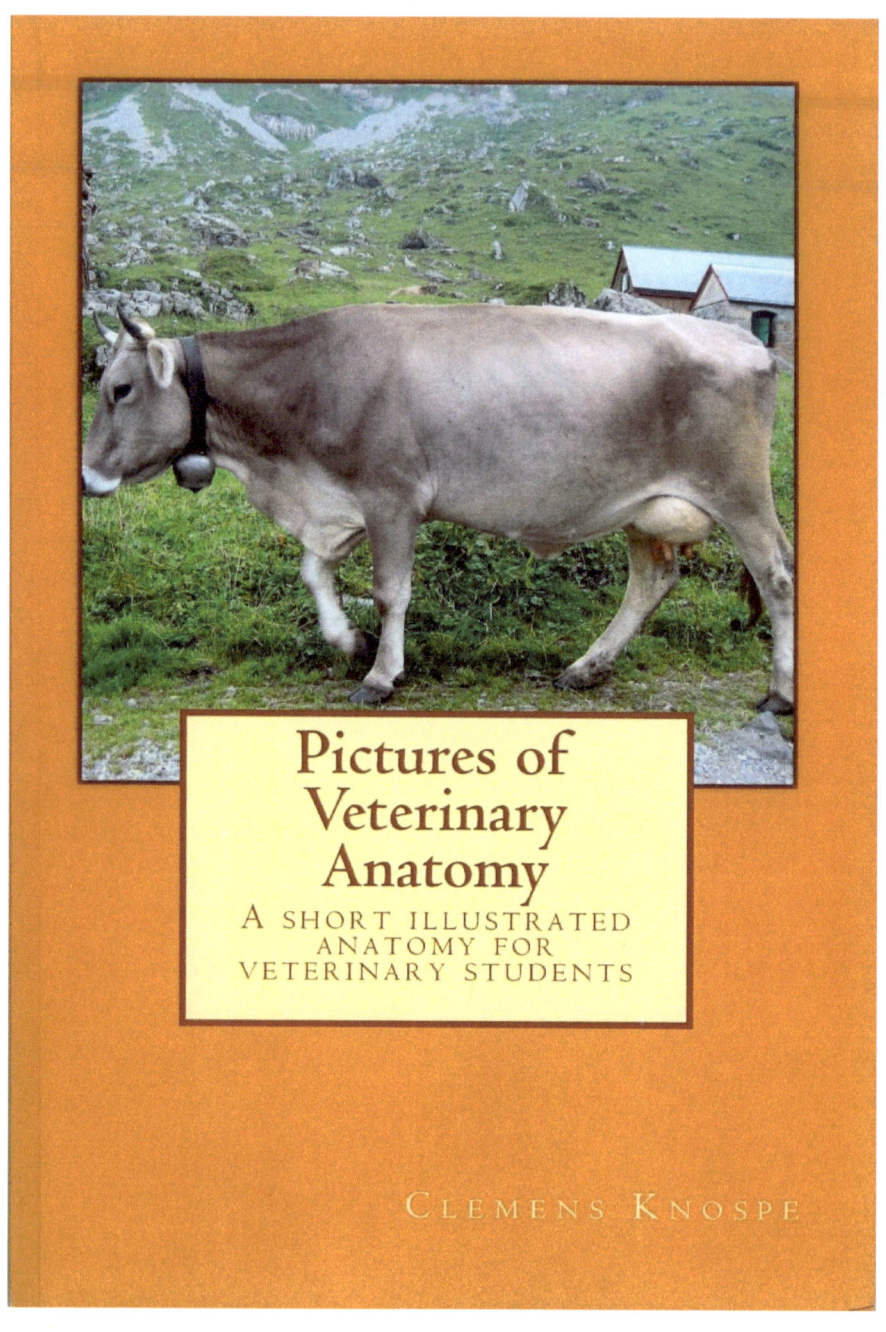

see also other books of Dr. Knospe

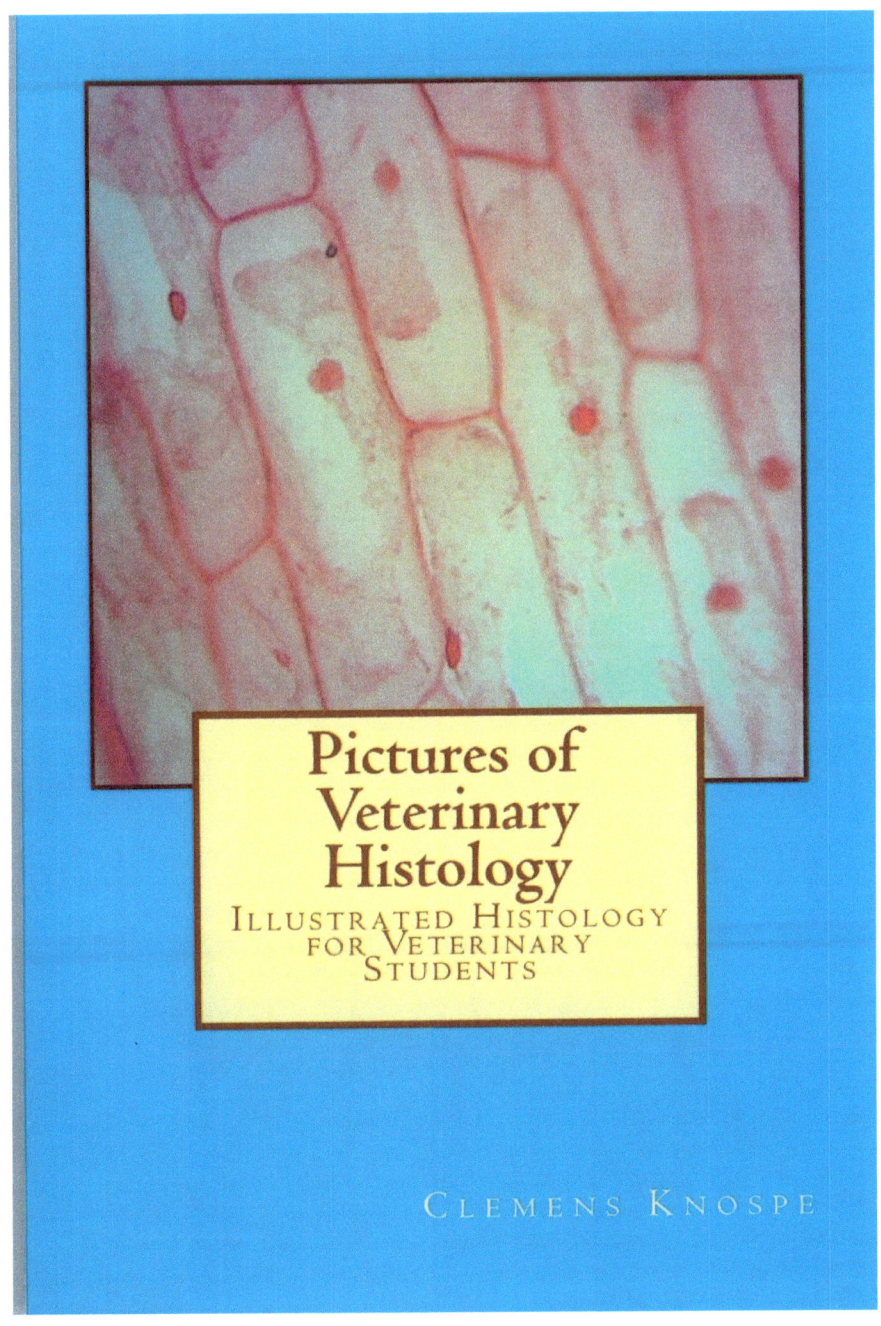

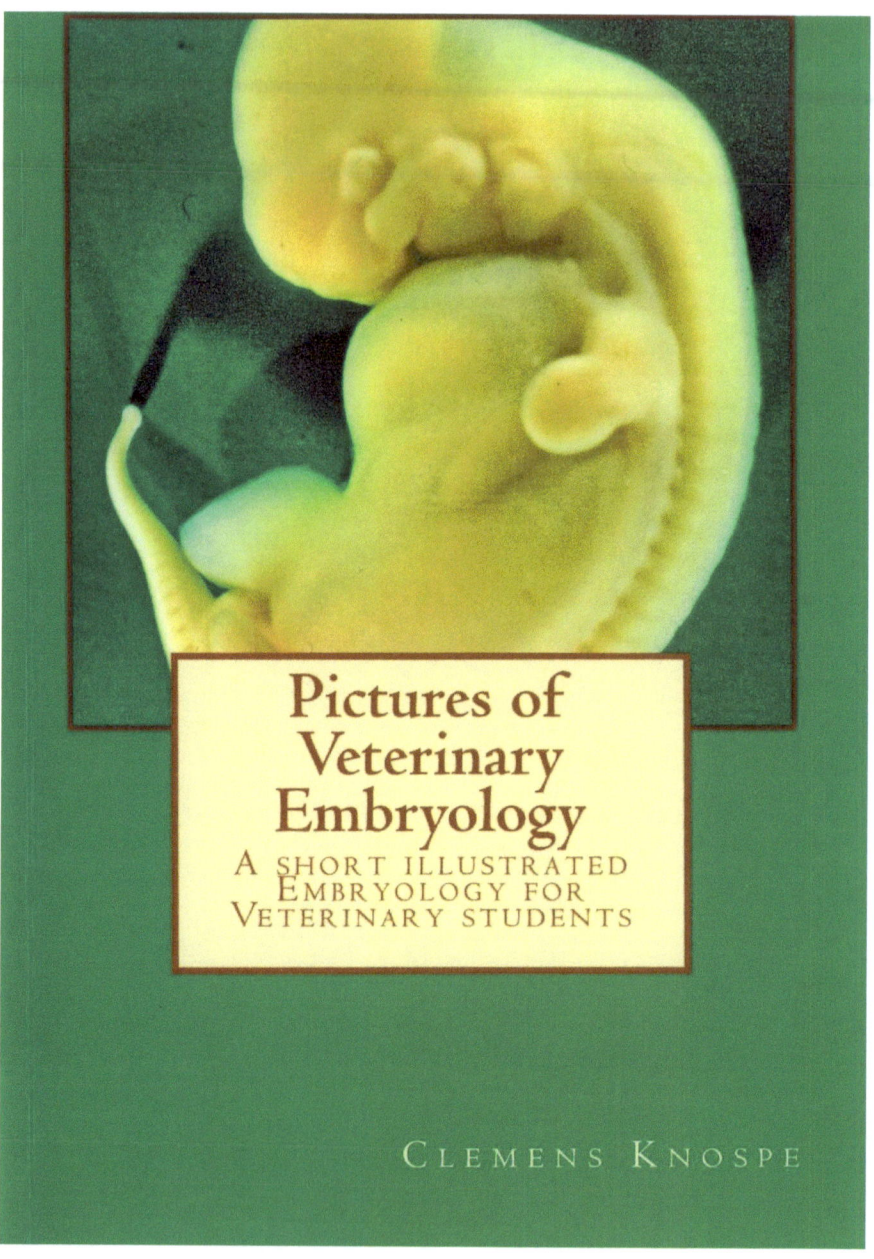

Dr. Clemens Knospe is Professor for Veterinary Anatomy, -Histology and -Embryology at the LMU Munich

www.ingramcontent.com/pod-product-compliance
Lightning Source LLC
Chambersburg PA
CBHW040808200526
45159CB00022B/56